W9-DDG-599

Confident Voices

The Nurses' Guide to Improving Communication & Creating Positive Workplaces

Author

Beth Boynton, RN, MS
www.bethboynton.com
www.confidentvoices.com

Editor

Bonnie Kerrick, RN, BSN
bdk123@maine.rr.com

Contributing Author

Judy Ringer, www.judyringer.com

Foreward

Joan Cusack-McGuirk, MA, BSN, NEA-BC
VP & CNO St. Luke's Cornwall Hospital
Newburgh/Cornwall, N.Y

Epilogue

Wanda Christie, MNSc, RN, OCN
Assistant Professor of Nursing
Arkansas Tech University, Russellville, AR

Photographer

Cheryl Brigham
www.cherations.com

Publishing Consultant

Jeffrey Elwood

Graphic Design

Joanne Muckenhoupt
www.redwinghill.com

Confident Voices

The Nurses' Guide to Improving Communication & Creating Positive Workplaces

CreateSpace, a DBA of On-Demand Publishing LLC, part of the Amazon group of companies.

ISBN 1440441707

EAN-13 9781440441707

Bonnie Kerrick, RN, BSN, Editor

Contributing authors, Judy Ringer , www.judyringer.com

Foreward by Joan Cusack-McGuirk, MA, BSN, NEA-BC

Epilogue by Wanda Christie, MNSc, RN, OCN

Cover art and design by Joanne Muchenhoupt, www.redwinghill.com

Publishing consultant, Jeffrey Elwood

Photography by Cheryl Brigham, www.cherations.com

Dedication

To Curran B. Russell, my very dear son and friend.

Table of Contents

Foreward

By Joan Cusack-McGuirk

This is not just another book on improving communication in order to create a healthy work environment. Boynton is able to capture key points around these topics: We need to pay attention, listen to what is being said, and her message is very clear....let's get back to basics.

Improving communication and creating a positive workplace is incorporating not only the science but the art of nursing. In *Confident Voices*, Boynton demonstrates both the science and the art and emphasizes that neither communication nor a healthy work environment can be achieved unless nurses and healthcare leaders engage in a collaborative participatory approach.

Boynton, through insightful identification of well-known scenarios, is able to link us to situations that we can all relate to. It is commendable that in the multifaceted climate in which we practice, she does not limit us to the narrow scope of healthcare but expands to the multiple expertises outside of nursing. It is through her storytelling, summaries of real life scenarios, that we can all relate and therefore advance to the next level. Although some may possess an innate ability for enhancing communication on developing positive work environments, there needs to be ongoing attention to the development of this talent. Boynton enhances our skill set to do so.

Boynton has a two-pronged approach. She speaks to those who recognize that building healthy work environments and enhancing communication is a skill to be cultivated. She also speaks to those who may not recognize that it takes practice, alertness, and a sincere desire to listen and pay attention. Boynton is able to drive some key points home by her ability to demonstrate real-life examples and strategies that all of us have experienced and can relate to. Boynton's ability to bring to life Daniel Goleman's concepts relative to emotional intelligence is quite meaningful.

As we continue to practice in a "whitewater" environment, this book could not come at a better time. When enhanced communication skills are key and a healthy work environment essential, it is critical to develop an environment and skills that will enhance practice, build relationships, and improve the quality of care to which we dedicate our life's work, our patients.

Joan Cusack-McGuirk, MA, BSN, NEA-BC
VP & CNO St. Luke's Cornwall Hospital
Newburgh/Cornwall, N.Y

Introduction

Congratulations on purchasing *Confident Voices: The Nurses' Guide to Improving Communication and Creating Positive Workplaces!* This stimulating and provocative book is guaranteed to get you thinking, talking, and acting in ways that will help you create positive workplaces!

In January of 2009, The Joint Commission's (TJC) new standards addressing behaviors that undermine a culture of safety go into effect.[1] Most simply put, the new performance expectations require hospitals/ organizations to have a "code of conduct" that defines appropriate and inappropriate behaviors and a process for managing inappropriate or disruptive ones. The timing is right and, despite the challenges of changing behavior, the fact that TJC is taking a leadership role in this direction is a cause for celebration!

Nurses have a tremendous potential to optimize healthcare systems! With over 3 million in the US, (12 million worldwide), we are healthcare's biggest workforce and are visible in just about any healthcare setting. By our very presence, we impact the culture of our workplaces. When we are thriving, we navigate incredible stress while providing highly skilled, compassionate, and rewarding service. The interconnectedness of quality, safety, creativity, and morale is enhanced beyond measure.

---

1 *The details of this new standard can be found on TJC's website by going to Sentinel Events, then Sentinal Event Alerts; Issue 40, Behaviors that undermine a culture of safety.*

Too often, however, we are not thriving. Staffing shortages and workplace violence are vicious negative cycles that add layers of frustration and stress. Instead of feeling empowered to change things, we feel hopeless and victimized. Resistance and burnout become expressions of our voices. We suffer in toxic workplaces that are harmful to our co-workers, our patients, and ourselves. Hardly the vision of nursing that many of us are seeking.

Confident Voices: The Nurses' Guide to Improving Communication and Creating Positive Workplaces provides a bridge to healthy professional relationships, positive workplaces, and creative problem solving. This short and compelling book integrates expertise from a variety of fields and applies it to nursing. Highlights from emotional intelligence, psychology, organizational behavior, leadership, communication, and conflict are masterfully crafted into a new lens. This new lens illuminates our current conditions in terms of relationships and organizational culture, allowing us to understand and evolve the dynamics of our workplaces.

> *How wonderful it is that nobody need wait a single moment before starting to improve the world.*
>
> **--Anne Frank**

The text is broken down into three main sections aimed at understanding the status quo, developing healthier skills and organizational cultures, and finally, integrating new practices into real nursing environments. It is filled with enlightening real-world stories, insights, and practical advice – all of which promote skills that lead to positive workplaces. Inspiring quotes, supplementary resources, and questions for discussion and reflection offer additional learning opportunities.

The value of this guide will vary with individuals and circumstances. Some learning, I believe, will take place immediately and some will take place over time with new experiences and observations. By shedding light on underlying issues which nurses face every day, *Confident Voices* creates a new foundation for interactions. Reading, reflecting, discussing, and practicing the content present an endless variety of applications. This book can be used for individual growth, study circles, or as a supplemental text in leadership, communication, conflict, and team-building instruction.

I believe that we can create more positive workplaces! We can do this by tapping into our own power and engaging in respectful and informed dialogues with each other. Your ideas, experiences, and insights are as much a part of building confident voices as the strategies I advocate.

Thank you for your commitment to the profession of nursing and your essential role in providing quality healthcare.

Beth

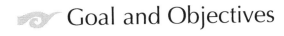 Goal and Objectives

Overarching Goal

To increase the positive impact nurses have on their careers, our profession, and the provision of safe, effective, patient-centered, timely, efficient, and equitable care.

Objectives

✓ To increase awareness and promote discussion among nurses and colleagues regarding ways individuals and organizations contribute to healthy vs. unhealthy work environments.

✓ To increase nurses' ability to be effective and respected communicators in healthcare organizations.

✓ To provide a resource for individuals, teachers, facilitators, and healthcare leaders that helps nurses improve communication skills and be active participants in the creation of positive workplaces.

✓ To increase awareness about the impact that communication and organizational culture have on nurses' ability to provide safe, effective, patient-centered, timely, efficient, and equitable care.

Part I: Understanding Workplace Dynamics

Overview

In the first four chapters, we will explore theories, research, and stories that expose and explain the current conditions in which many nurses work. Gaining a better understanding of the individual and organizational factors that contribute to toxic workplaces is important for several reasons. It gives us a reality check about where we are now, offers a powerful incentive to change, and helps solidify a commitment to creating positive workplaces. Unhealthy workplace dynamics are not present in all nurse practice settings, but sadly, they are ingrained in the status quo of many. These environments are not acceptable! The more we can identify and articulate inappropriate behavior, disruptive conduct, or toxic organizational cultures, the more empowered we will be for transforming our workplaces.

Chapter One

Toxic Workplaces and the Need for Change

Nurses are pivotal players in major issues such as patient safety and quality of care, recruitment, retention, and workplace violence. In various workshops and courses I teach on effective communication and conflict, I hear nurses say over and over: "Our healthcare system is broken and too complicated to fix." "What can nurses realistically do?" "We are the most trusted and visible workforce in healthcare; where is our power?" "Where are our voices?"

Ruth's Story

> I have been an RN for 31 years and began to experience abuse at work 28 years ago from a new young doctor (I'll call him Dr. X), who was only a year older than I. We both still work at the same small rural hospital in New England, and things between us have barely improved since. The initial interaction occurred when I was working in the Special Care Unit. A patient of his had become unconscious, due to a lidocaine drip (no pumps back then). Dr X ran into the unit and screamed at me, "What the hell did you do to my patient?" With him it was, and still remains, not so much the words he uses but the scathing, hateful way he says them.

Nurses are smart people who have successfully completed a rigorous academic and clinical program. I had a BS in biochemistry before going to nursing school and was amazed at the level of difficulty the nursing curriculum presented. We deal with sophisticated scientific principles and technology, endless interruptions, shifting priorities, stressful dynamics, excessive workloads, emotional stress, conflicting agendas, continuous change, and infinite urgent responsibilities. It is extraordinarily challenging work – intellectually, emotionally, and physically.

However, as I have developed my expertise in communication, conflict, team building, and leadership, I have observed two widespread issues. One is that nurses (as well as other healthcare professionals), are not always the most effective communicators, and, two, the environments we work in are often toxic.

> *In organizations, real power and energy is generated through relationships. The things we fear most in organizations—fluctuations, disturbances, imbalances—are the primary sources of creativity.*
>
> **--Margaret J. Wheatley**

With more than twenty years of experience as a nurse, organizational development consultant, and teacher, I am convinced that problems with communication and organizational culture are at the heart of many healthcare issues. As I see it, our communication patterns and the environments we work in arise from, and are reinforced by, individual and organizational behaviors.

The Joint Commission (TJC) has advised healthcare organizations to provide assertiveness training, flatten hierarchies, and promote a zero tolerance for abuse.[2] Consider how revealing these recommendations are. Assertiveness training addresses passive, passive-aggressive, and aggressive behaviors; flattening hierarchies is a solution for unproductive or inappropriate uses of power; and having a clear standard for not tolerating abuse is a strategy that recognizes and begins to deal with abuse in the environments where nurses work.

Ruth's Story continued

> Over the years, I have complained to my various supervisors about Dr X. Some ignored or dismissed my concerns. Any advice I did get, such as "Tell him to go f--- himself," was unprofessional and totally inappropriate. And I was not the only one to voice my concern; dozens of people from lab techs to X-ray techs to office workers have also complained about him, but nothing was ever done. The hospital administration has let him get away with this abusive behavior for close to 30 years.

Stories of nurses who "eat their young," abusive physicians, and toxic workplaces are commonplace throughout the healthcare system. Such stories are evidence of dysfunctional conflicts, which are a counterproductive part of our healthcare culture. Changing these workplace dynamics will be challenging, but not impossible. We can begin the process by promoting three key principles: respectful listening, speaking up assertively, and creating a safe environment. I believe that if we do not consistently address these foundational principles, we will

---

2 The Joint Commission Guide to Improving Staff Communication, *The Joint Commission Resources, 2005*

undermine the results of every other problem-solving intervention we apply!

Organizational leaders and nurses need to simultaneously establish, insist on, and follow healthy standards for communicating and working together. We don't need to become great friends or change personalities, but we do need effective communication skills and supportive organizational cultures so that our interactions are respectful, responsible, and effective. This book lays the foundation for this work.

The changes I recommend here are demanding because they require new behaviors. We need to think, reflect, discuss, and practice new ideas about our working selves and our relationships.

> *Nobody is going to come save you, that's your job. Save yourself. The object is not for them to like you, the object is for them to listen to you. Nobody knows what you want except you. And nobody will be as sorry as you if you don't get it.*
>
> **--Lillian Hellman**

Ruth's Story continued

Sometimes when I have to work with Dr. X, I become so anxious that I get diarrhea. I get flustered and can't think straight, and I believe he knows it. I find myself giving second-rate nursing care because I'm afraid to go to him with questions about orders or other patient-care issues.

When I see his car in the parking lot or hear his voice on the unit, I feel a sense of dread.

Recently, at a workshop on listening, a Chief Nursing Officer, (CNO) and Chief Finance Officer, (CFO) were arguing over the CFO's reference to MDs as a resource regarding issues involving their new computerized medical record system. The CNO objected to the CFO's use of the MDs, insisting that he include other healthcare providers. The CFO made a disapproving face and stated that when he said "MDs" he meant all clinical people.

The CNO seemed to feel that the CFO's comments were excluding nurses and others from also being resources for addressing the computerized system and was trying to advocate for her staff and perhaps, her profession. The CFO believed that he was including nurses in his use of the term MDs and seemed frustrated that the CNO would raise an issue about this.

Their communication efforts quickly disintegrated into interrupting each other and defending their own positions.

In this example, these two senior managers have a wealth of education, experience, and knowledge to draw from, but their energy is caught up in a struggle to be heard. The chances for creative problem solving are slim until these two professionals can listen to and respect each other's perspective.

Think about how the energy might shift if the CNO could express her frustrations about herself and staff feeling excluded and ask the CFO to be mindful of his use of the term MDs, and if the CFO would validate her perspective and make an effort to be more careful with his language.

Doesn't it seem likely that these efforts would help to build kinder, more respectful work relationships and, from these new relationships, create more productive conversations and strategies about the new system? I believe that if this CNO would speak up with ownership and if this CFO would practice effective listening, they could come up with better ideas and, ultimately, more investment in successful outcomes!

Summary

The kind of dynamic that is portrayed in Ruth's story, as well as that between the CNO and CFO, are pervasive and destructive. In Ruth's scenario, we see how intimidating treatment, lack of confidence, and unresponsive administration all contribute to a miserable situation for the nurse and set the stage for unsafe care. She might delay contacting the doctor or avoid running into him on the floor. With the CNO and CFO, I wonder how effectively they are working together on senior level issues that impact financial and nursing operations.

Within the dynamics of these relationships, opportunities for communicating about patient status or related concerns, collaborative problem-solving, and creativity are lost. They are tricky to measure, subtle at times, and very complicated, if not impossible to recover. Nevertheless, stressed or toxic relationships among healthcare professionals are not uncommon. Further, they directly or indirectly impact the healthcare system in a variety of ways including, but not limited to, quality, safety, and job satisfaction. Sometimes the results are catastrophic. These toxic dynamics are not OK.

In addition to TJC's new conduct standard, the ideas presented here are in sync with the goals promoted by the Institute of Medicine's Committee on Quality of Healthcare in America for safe, effective, patient-centered, timely, efficient, and equitable care.[3] Eventually, these new ways of "being at work" will require growth, learning, and commitment from healthcare workers at all levels and from all specialties. Nurses can champion this work NOW!

---

3 *Committee on Quality of Healthcare in America, Institute of Medicine. 2001.* Crossing the Quality Chasm: A New Health System for the 21st Century. *Washington, DC: National Academy Press.*

Discussion Questions

1. How would you describe Ruth's relationship with Dr. X?

2. How do you think this relationship contributes to her ability to provide professional nursing care?

3. How do you think patients and/or family members might interpret the dynamics between Ruth and Dr. X?

4. Do you think the hospital administrators in Ruth's story contribute to the dynamic between Ruth and Dr. X? If so, how?

5. Can you think of any problems in healthcare today that are not impacted by toxic relationships?

Reflection Questions

1. Have you ever felt intimidated by a physician, nurse, or administrative leader? If so, describe an example of an interaction with this person.

2. How do you think this affected or affects you personally and professionally?

3. Have you ever shared this experience with a colleague? What was his/her response?

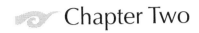 Chapter Two

Individuals and Relationships at Work

In this chapter, we will review some familiar theories, add some highlights from emotional intelligence and organizational behavior, and begin to look at how these theories can help us understand some of our own needs, reactions, and values – especially with respect to our behaviors and relationships at work. Although most of this book uses real-world scenarios and practical advice, this theoretical foundation will set the stage for a deeper level of understanding regarding the work we need to do.

In school and continuing education classes, we have studied concepts from psychology, education, and sociology. Often our learning is focused on how the information can help us understand patients' needs, reactions, and values, which helps us be more understanding and effective in caring for them. We can turn to many of the same theories for help in understanding and taking care of ourselves.

Maslow's Hierarchy of Needs

Abraham Maslow is well known for his ideas on human motivation, and his work has evolved over the years to include eight levels of progressive needs:[4]

1. **Physiological**: hunger, thirst, bodily comforts, etc.

2. **Safety/security**: out of danger

---

4 Maslow, A., & Lowery, R. (Ed.). (1998). Toward a Psychology of Being (3rd ed.). New York: Wiley & Sons.

3. **Belonging and love**: affiliate with others, be accepted

4. **Esteem**: to achieve, be competent, gain approval and recognition

5. **Cognitive**: to know, to understand, and explore

6. **Aesthetic**: symmetry, order, and beauty

7. **Self-actualization:** to find self-fulfillment and realize one's potential

8. **Self-transcendence:** to connect to something beyond the ego or to help others find self-fulfillment and realize their potential

In day-to-day work environments, nurses must focus on patient needs. Requests to meet these needs may come from patients, doctors, families, administrators, and other healthcare professionals. This may be part of the reason why many of us are more adept at identifying and addressing the needs of others rather than our own.

To some extent, this is the nature of the job, and yet, our needs are important too. Sometimes healthcare organizations seem to exploit the care-giving role of nurses, and sometimes, I think we do this to ourselves.

Years ago, as a med-surg staff RN at a busy teaching hospital, I rarely took meal breaks. In retrospect, I believe that some of this was because I didn't want to ask for help, didn't want to interrupt the flow of my work, and/or didn't really think I needed to take a break. I also believe that, given my patient assignment, I would not have been able to get my work done in time or would have had to cut corners in some way.

Organizationally, there are often expectations of excessive workloads, unrealistic estimations of the time required to follow procedure and communicate effectively, and an under appreciation of the stressors involved as nurses strive to carry out the physical, emotional, and intellectual challenges of providing safe, quality nursing care.

Individually, we may have a hard time saying "No," experience satisfaction from "saving the day," and/or put insidious pressure on colleagues to make sacrifices according to some unwritten nursing standard. Sometimes it seems that, rather than set limits and respect other nurses who do, we become martyrs and resent our colleagues when they try to set healthier limits.

If we are willing to look at both the organizational and individual factors that are contributing to toxic work environments, we will be much more empowered to create positive workplaces.

McGregor's Theories X and Y

In Douglas McGregor's *The Human Side of Enterprise,* he describes two management philosophies which are closely tied to motivation.[5] According to McGregor, leaders who believe in **Theory X** assume that people:

✓ Have a genuine distaste for work.

✓ Must be prodded, coerced, or threatened to work because it is so unpleasant.

✓ Prefer to be closely supervised.

✓ Avoid as much responsibility as they can.

---

5 *McGregor, D. (1960). The Human Side of Enterprise, New York: Harper & Row.*

23

✓ Have little ambition.

✓ Value security above all else.

Leaders who follow **Theory Y**, McGregor advises, assume that people:

✓ Want to work because work is natural.

✓ Will exercise self-control if they are committed to the results to be achieved by their efforts.

✓ Will be motivated to achieve goals if they value those goals.

✓ Share imagination and creativity, traits that are not limited solely to management.

✓ Are boxed-in by bureaucratic job descriptions and are capable of realizing more potential than they are typically given a chance to realize.

Although I have observed a few employees who seem to fit the assumptions of Theory X, this is often the result of poor relationships and/or a feeling of powerlessness or power struggles with management. During my years as an occupational health nurse, I saw how employees respond when they are coerced or dominated. Those who are not treated respectfully will exhibit behaviors consistent with Theory X. Of course, poor treatment may have been experienced at a previous job or in a family situation, which makes the cause-and-effect of behavior more complex.

I have seen employees with workers compensation injuries who, if they have a say in their light duty work and are generally happy in their job, will get back to work much earlier and with minimal, if any, case management. Conversely, if an employee is not happy in her/his job or there is a supervisory conflict and/or mindset to force him/her back to work, the complications and case management needs rise sharply. Employees who have little voice in their return to work may use being injured as if it is their only source of power.

A simple invitation for employee input regarding any problem can make the difference between a collaborative effort and a power struggle. A collaborative approach shows respect, promotes

> *Know that although in the eternal scheme of things you are small, you are also unique and irreplaceable, as are all your fellow humans everywhere in the world.*
>
> **--Margaret Laurence**

buy-in, and taps into an employee's ideas. Power struggles, on the other hand, lack respect, promote resistance, and eliminate the employee as a resource. Such power struggles reflect enormous drains on an organization's resources in terms of time, money, and emotional energy.

Chris Argyris, PhD: When Passivity and Dependence are Conditions at Work

What happens when professionals become frustrated in cultures where supervisors maintain tight controls over their employees? Chris Argyris, PhD, one of the pioneer theorists of organizational behavior, believes that the consequences of a controlling management result in passivity and dependence. He describes six responses that employees may have when faced with overly controlling management.

- ✓ They withdraw through chronic absenteeism or simply by quitting.

- ✓ They stay on the job, but withdraw psychologically, becoming indifferent, passive, and apathetic.

- ✓ They resist by restricting output, or engaging in deception, featherbedding, or sabotage.

- ✓ They try to climb the hierarchy to better jobs.

- ✓ They form groups (such as labor unions) to redress the power imbalance.

- ✓ They socialize their children to believe that work is unrewarding and hopes for advancement are slim.

When I first read this list, I was amazed to make connections with some of my own behaviors as well as those of some of my colleagues. Over the course of my career, I have left two positions (one as a staff nurse and one as a clinical director), because of frustration and feelings of powerlessness. I know I wasn't a perfect employee, but I was a sharp and caring nurse in both positions. I believe that individuals at all levels want to be respected and heard. It is part of being human.

Optimism

In Daniel Goleman's popular book *Emotional Intelligence*, he compares optimism to hope and describes a frame of mind that anticipates that everything will turn out OK even though problems may occur.[6] From the standpoint of emotional intelligence, he indicates that optimism is a quality that keeps people from falling into hopelessness, apathy, or despair. He further indicates that inborn temperament and personal experience can contribute to a person's sense of optimism or hope as well as to feelings of helplessness or despair. According to Goleman, "self-efficacy" is a term that psychologists use to describe one's sense of mastery over, and ability to cope with, setbacks in one's life. Given these thoughts, it seems that having a sense of power in life, or for our purposes, at work, is closely tied to motivation. It follows from Goleman's theories that organizations have opportunities to build optimism or despair.

> *The future belongs to those who believe in the beauty of their dreams.*
>
> **--Eleanor Roosevelt**

Motivation

There are all sorts of theories about motivation. From a common sense vantage point, we already know that changing behavior is difficult! It is also generally accepted that accomplishing any change is much more likely when the individuals involved are invested in the outcome.

---

6 *Goleman, D. (1995). Emotional Intelligence: Why it Can Matter More than IQ. New York, NY: Bantam Books.*

Understanding what makes people behave or perform in certain ways has implications for individuals as well as leaders. As nursing professionals, we are often challenged to find ways to influence patients' behaviors in an effort to improve (or empower them to improve), their well-being. As individuals, we are often looking for help with reaching personal goals, such as continuing education, saving money, or losing weight. In the business world, developing strategies that motivate employees to meet goals and accomplish the organizational mission are top priorities. Author Quint Studer, in his book, *Hardwiring Excellence*, focuses on building positive attitudes in hospitals and suggests that healthcare personnel are already highly motivated.[7]

It stands to reason that when individuals have clarity about what they want and need and when organizations are clear about goals, mission, and vision, the potential for effective intrinsic and extrinsic motivation increase sharply and, with it, successful outcomes.

Margaret J. Wheatley, management professor and organizational theorist, writes about motivation and its connection to collaborative experiences in the third edition of her book, *Leadership and the New Science*.[8] In her opinion, "Motivation for individual change is not a response to a bosses' demand or personal need for self-improvement." She explains that being part of a collaborative process allows individuals to see how their own behaviors contribute to the team. This leads to a personal decision to change in order to help the team be more effective.

---

7 *Studer, Q. (2003).* Hardwiring Excellence. *Gulf Breeze, FL: Fire Starter Publishing.*

8 *Wheatley, Margaret J.,* Leadership and the New Science, *2006, San Francisco, CA, Berret-Koehler Publishers.*

I believe that Dr. Wheatley is illuminating a core human desire that speaks to our ability to be part of a team and find joy in contributing our own gifts. Speaking up and listening respectfully are integral components of this collaborative process. Consequently, the focus of this book on building and supporting those skills is related to optimizing motivation. Imagine how powerful and productive a unit could be when individual and organizational desires are aligned, authentic, and combined with interactions that are healthy!

Relationship Power

The inherent qualities, such as optimism and motivation that individuals bring to and/or develop in the workplace, become even more significant when we consider how they inform our relationships and how relationships can make or break organizations. Wheatley writes about relationships and power: "What gives power its charge, positive or negative, is the nature of the relationship. When power is shared in such workplace redesigns as participative management and self-managed teams, positive creative power abounds."

> *Never doubt that a small group of thoughtful, committed citizens can change the world. Indeed, it is the only thing that can.*
>
> **--Margaret Mead**

Sometimes I hear healthcare administration students complaining that self-managed teams are a disaster and lead to more frustration and problems than they are worth. They tell me that employees are unreliable, overly dependent on management intervention, and often complain about their colleagues. I challenge them to consider the quality

29

of relationships and the communication culture they are working in. Do people feel free to give honest feedback and feel safe hearing it? Are expectations and roles clear or at least clear enough? Does the staff have the resources and skills they need to realistically meet the goals? When self-managed teams fail, it is tempting to conclude that they don't work. It is more difficult to explore these questions and consider how the team-building process and organizational supports may have influenced the outcome.

Summary

How we behave at work and interact with colleagues is closely tied to our sense of self and the supports available to us. Both can be major sources of creativity or destruction.

Communication is a primary way in which we express ourselves and define to others who we are. It is a fundamental part of how we develop our relationships and explains why related skills are so important and incredibly complex. When the foundations of relationships are based on solid values such as trust, respect, and kindness, the creative problem solving that can emerge has enormous ramifications for quality of care, job satisfaction, and related healthcare issues.

Backbiting, resistance to change, dismissing others, or withholding ideas are all negative behaviors that can undermine constructive communication at work. They are unproductive, and are, too often, inappropriate expressions of what we want, need, think, or feel.

It makes sense that when people have a voice in their work, they are motivated by their own will and are more likely to develop authentic relationships. Looking for ways to practice and encourage nurses to have a voice – not only for reporting clinical issues, but to add creative ideas, set limits, give and receive feedback – should be an individual and organizational priority for healthcare systems.

I know that creating systems with solid values is a daunting process. It will take time, experience, resources, and consistent, devoted individuals and leaders who are committed to the process.

While we are developing confident voices and positive workplaces, we can implement a practical measure now by creating a standard of communication that is respectful. I can't make you respect me, but I can insist upon respectful treatment. Organizations can train, promote, and enforce the same.

I believe that this is a realistic and no-nonsense business strategy that healthcare systems must embark on. It is a pathway to healthier relationships and can evolve even in the midst of dysfunction. The stakes are high.

In April 2006, officials with the Health Resources and Services Administration (HRSA) released projections that the nation's nursing shortage would grow to more than one million nurses by the year 2020. In the report "What is Behind HRSA's Projected Supply, Demand, and Shortage of Registered Nurses?" analysts show that all 50 states will experience a shortage of nurses to varying degrees by the year 2015.

Our voices are expressions of personal and professional power. When confident, we are open to other perspectives, listen respectfully, build authentic relationships, and are able to advocate for ourselves and our patients. We deserve to be treated respectfully and must play an active role in making that happen.

Discussion Questions

1. Have you ever been part of a self-managed team? What factors contributed to the successes or challenges of this experience?

2. What ideas do you have to increase self-efficacy among nurses in general? Can you think of any organizational efforts that would help?

3. Which of my needs do you think I was honoring when I was a staff nurse skipping meal breaks? Was I ignoring any?

4. Have you ever noticed a nurse getting angry or resentful at another when s/he tried to make her/his own needs a priority, such as refusing to come in on a day off or to work overtime? What do you think might be going on here?

5. Consider two nurse managers: one who believes in Theory X and the other, Theory Y. How might each of these managers approach a situation where a staff nurse was demonstrating a pattern of being late to work? How do you think the staff nurse might respond to these different approaches?

Reflection Questions

1. What led you to nursing as a career? Does your work as a nurse help to meet any of these needs for you?

2. Can you think of a situation at work where you did or did not share an idea or concern?

3. Which assumptions from Theory X and/or Y do you find motivating? How about assumptions that seem de-motivating?

4. What are the top three things that motivate you to provide top-notch nursing care?

Chapter Three

Organizational Culture

Individual and organizational behaviors are not really separate phenomena. We impact our work environment, and our work environment impacts us. On some level, both impact the care we give. In this chapter, we will focus on some highlights about organizational culture that can simply be stated as the way the people in an organization do things. Later, in chapter seven, we'll look more closely at how we can create safe environments where healthcare professionals and services can thrive.

How employees dress, their understanding and beliefs in the mission and vision, and how they approach conflict are all integrated into an organization's culture. Understanding the organizational culture becomes more complicated when we consider the many variables that contribute to it. Interpersonal skills, professional practices, diversity, nature of the work, trust, and leadership expectations are all factors that become part of an organization's culture.

All members of an organization contribute to the culture by following or challenging the status quo. Depending on power and position, individuals may have varying amounts of influence on changing or maintaining the culture. For some individuals to stay in an organization, the culture may require them to change their behavior. They may adapt outwardly, but if the culture is contrary to their values, they may face constant turmoil. In other situations, individuals may leave the organization because they are not compatible with the culture.

Ideally, an organization's culture will support the people and practices that are necessary to accomplish its mission and vision.

As nurses, I believe that efforts aimed at improving our workplaces will have a positive impact on safety, quality, and staffing. Keep in mind that, as overwhelming this may seem, changing the status quo is a process in which we can all play a part. As we develop confident voices, individually and collectively, our influence will grow.

Types of Organizational Culture

There are several theories regarding types of organizational culture. We will focus on one reviewed in the book, *Organizational Behavior Key Concepts, Skills, & Best Practices.*[9] Here, authors Kinicki and Kreitner describe three types of organizational culture based on work done by Cooke, R. A. and Szumal, J.L.[10] These three cultures are: Constructive, Passive-defensive, and Aggressive-defensive. Each culture has a set of defining characteristics and normative beliefs around expected behaviors and approaches to work associated with it. Highlights from each of these types are listed below. Consider the organizations and units you have worked in as you read about these cultures.

A Constructive culture is one that values achievement, self-actualizing, humanistic-encouraging, and affiliative behaviors. Characteristics that this type of culture values include:

---

9 Organizational Behavior: Key Concepts, Skills & Best Practices, *Kinicki, Angelo and Kreitner, Robert, McGraw-Hill/ Irwin, New York, NY, (2008).*

10 *"Measuring Normative Beliefs and Shared Behavioral Expectations in Organizations: The Reliability and Validity of the Organizational Cultural Inventory."* Psychological Reports, 1993, Vol 72, pg 1299-1330.

- ✓ Members who enthusiastically set and work towards their own goals.

- ✓ Members who set challenging, but realistic goals.

- ✓ Creativity.

- ✓ Quality over quantity.

- ✓ Accomplishment of tasks and individual growth.

- ✓ Participatory leadership.

- ✓ Supportive, constructive, friendly, open, and sensitive interpersonal relationships.

A **Passive-defensive culture** is one that values approval, dependent, avoidant, and conventional approaches to work. Characteristics that this type of culture values include:

- ✓ Avoidance of conflicts.

- ✓ Pleasant, even if superficial, relationships.

- ✓ Members who agree with, and seek approval from, each other.

- ✓ Conservative, traditional, hierarchal, bureaucratic, and non-participatory leadership.

- ✓ Members who conform, follow the rules, and make a good impression.

✓ A negative reward system which leads members to blame others and avoid possibility for being blamed, while ignoring successes.

A Passive-aggressive culture is one that values dominant, oppositional, competitive, and perfectionist approaches to work. Characteristics that this type of culture values include:

✓ Members who are critical of and/or oppose others.

✓ Members are rewarded for taking charge, controlling subordinates, and being controlled by superiors.

✓ Positional authority.

✓ Winning and outperforming others leads to job security and status.

✓ Perfection, persistence, and hard work.

✓ Members avoid making mistakes, keep track of everything, work long hours, and narrowly define goals.

A constructive culture seems like a great vision to work towards, and, in fact, describes a spirit of collaboration that many healthcare systems are working towards. However, in my experience, many teams and organizations seem to have more qualities found in the passive-defensive and aggressive-defensive cultures.

To complicate matters, there are times when characteristics from passive-defensive and passive-aggressive cultures may contribute to a positive healthcare workplace. Avoiding conflict, hierarchal structures, perfection, persistence, and hard work are often appropriate and constructive. The tricky parts are deciding when we need what and how to maintain respectful dynamics across the board. Avoiding a conflict about disruptive behavior during a code is a wise strategy. Addressing it assertively shortly after and preventing future incidents is equally important.

Cultures of Blame

What happens when we have a tendency to blame others when things go wrong in clinical situations? In his article "Ending the Blame Game Creating & Sustaining a Blame-Free Culture: A Foundation for Process Improvement,"[11] Author Manoj Pawar, MD, MMM, describes how a culture of blame interferes with a healthcare organization's goals around quality, service, and innovation. Although his article is aimed at physician leaders, there is much that can be applied across-the-board to nurses as leaders and role models. Here is a summary of his six reasons that describe how blame interferes with organizational success:

- ✓ It has a negative emotional context, which instills fear, anger, and resentment leading to dysfunctional relationships and poor morale.

- ✓ It shifts energy and focus towards self-preservation – attacking, and defending rather than understanding and learning.

- ✓ It causes biases for holding onto one's perspective and position, which limits potential for innovation and improvement.

---

11 *"Ending the Blame Game Creating & Sustaining a Blame-Free Culture: A Foundation for Process Improvement," Manoj Pawar, MD, MMM, The Physician Executive, July • August 2007, pg 12-14.*

✓ It inhibits creativity, because people become fearful and are more likely to operate from a protective and safe stance rather than being open and curious.

✓ It is expensive in terms of quality, service failures, staff turnover, customer satisfaction, morale, waste, and lost opportunity.

✓ It can kill, because it inhibits honest speaking out.

Respectful communication is an integral part of accountability and is severely limited by cultures of blame. This book works to simultaneously address building communication skills for nurses and organizational cultures that will support them. We must be able to own our part in a mistake and feel safe in doing so.

This major undertaking is complicated by regulations, fears of litigation, scope of practice, staffing ratios, and financial issues. I do not pretend to think that effective communication will magically solve these concerns, but I strongly believe that it will provide a healthier foundation for discovering better ways to address them.

Peter Senge and the Learning Organization

Peter Senge, well known in the business world, defines learning organizations in his book, *The Fifth Discipline. The art and practice of the learning organization,*[12] as "...organizations where people continually expand their capacity to create the results they truly desire, where new and expansive patterns of thinking are nurtured, where collective

---

12 *Senge, P. M. (1990)* The Fifth Discipline: The art and practice of the learning organization, *London: Random House.*

aspiration is set free, and where people are continually learning to see the whole together."

In this type of organization, there is a culture of learning that contrasts sharply with the culture of blame discussed earlier. Consider how a different list might evolve if the culture supported learning rather than blame.

- ✓ The emotional context becomes one of respect, acceptance, and safety, promoting functional relationships and improving morale.

- ✓ Energy is focused on understanding and learning.

- ✓ People are more open to seeing new and different perspectives, allowing for innovation and improvement.

- ✓ Creativity is enhanced by open minds and curious thinking.

- ✓ Financial savings are realized in terms of consistent quality, decreased failures, turnover, waste, and lost opportunity, with increases in morale and customer satisfaction.

- ✓ Fewer medical errors occur because people are not afraid to speak up.

June Fabre, RN, MBA, and Smart Nursing

In her book, *Smart Nursing*,[13] June Fabre describes seven core values and ten guiding principles that form the foundation for quality healthcare and positive workplaces.

The seven core values of Smart Nursing:

1. Caring

2. Respect

3. Simplicity

4. Flexibility

5. Integrity

6. Professional culture

7. Communication

The ten guiding principles of Smart Health Care Management:

1. Nurses are an essential part of a healthcare facility's investment.

2. Systems problems prevent nurses from performing at their full professional capacity.

---

13 *June Fabre, MBA, RNC,* Smart Nursing: Nurse Retention & Patient Safety Improvement Strategies, *Second Edition, 2008, New York, NY, Springer Publishing Company.*

3. Restoring the value of nursing by considering nurses as assets and treating them as valued professionals maximizes the return on an organization's human resource investment.

4. Organizations that provide environments where nurses can perform at their best attract and retain the best people.

5. Leaders and managers are more effective when they build strong relationships with their staff.

6. Long-term strategies, such as effective communication and staff-friendly cultures, enable organizations to achieve the best results.

7. Combining sound clinical practices with ethical business actions produces the safest and most cost-effective patient care.

8. Positive relationships among healthcare professionals generate energy and raise productivity.

9. Clinical nurses who can make decisions at the patient level save management time and increase patient satisfaction.

10. Individuals who embrace lifelong learning develop the ability to thrive in a rapidly changing world.

June's book is a great resource for explaining how nurses and organizations can work together to improve patient care and work environments with many cost-effective and practical strategies.

Summary

The organizational cultures that nurses work in make a significant difference in quality of care they give and how they feel at the end of the day. Leaders from all disciplines and staff nurses from all specialties are instrumental in creating cultures that support or hinder a sense of confidence.

A supportive environment is one where listening and respect are trusted norms. This means that, in addition to offering standardized assertiveness training, organizations must look for ways to respect and affirm what nurses need, want, and think.

> *People don't resist change. They resist being changed.*
>
> **--Peter M. Senge**

Although healthcare leaders have more power to initiate, educate. and enforce changes, individual nurses can also champion a positive culture by practicing, discussing, and reflecting on new ways of "being at work." As you will see throughout this book, there are many opportunities for organizations and/or committed professionals to help nurses gain confidence in expressing their concerns, setting limits, and sharing feedback.

Organizations that support and respect nursing staff will be workplaces where nurses thrive. When nurses can be clear about the support they need and the ways they deserve to be treated, organizations will know what they need to do to cultivate the best nursing staff.

In this light, we can begin to see the interdependence of staff and leaders in building a culture where speaking up and respectful listening are equally emphasized.

Leaders who understand the complexity involved in this evolution and work to help nurses develop awareness and skills along theses lines will be contributing beyond measure to healthier staff, more collaborative systems and safer, higher quality and more cost effective care.

Discussion Questions

1. Which characteristics of each culture do you think play a positive role in nurse practice settings?   What examples can you think of that support your opinion? Could any of these also play a toxic role?

2. Which characteristics of each culture involve some aspect of communication?

3. What ideas do you have for leaders who want to shift from a passive-defensive culture to a constructive one? How about from a passive-aggressive culture?

Reflection Questions

1. How would you describe the culture at your workplace?

2. What adjectives would you use to describe an ideal work culture for you?

3. What kind of training would you need to be an active participant in the ideal culture?

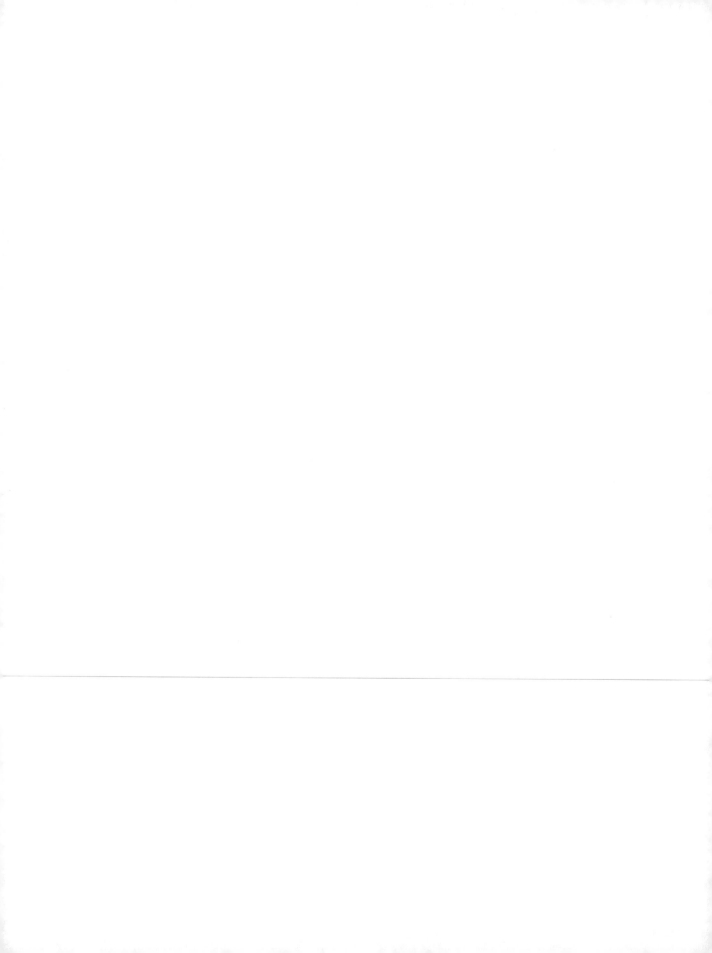

Chapter Four

Workplace Violence

Dorrie's Story

Over my 20-year career as a pediatric and community health nurse, I always managed to make relationships with staff and physicians work in order to provide the best possible care. Sometimes I swallowed my pride, but I realized that working in healthcare was extremely stressful for all us.

Aggression is the most common behavior used by many organizations, a nearly invisible medium that influences all decisions and actions.

--Margaret J. Wheatley

✓ Verbal abuse contributes to up to 24% of staff turnover and 42% of nurse administrator turnover. More staggering is the report that 60% of new-to-practice nurses leave their first professional position within six months because of lateral (horizontal) violence; 20% of these new-to-practice nurses leave the profession forever (Hurley, J. 2006).[14]

---

14 Hurley, J., *"Nurse-to-Nurse Horizontal Violence: Recognizing it and Preventing it."* NSNA Imprint. *September/October 2006.*

Dorrie's Story continued

I accepted that it was part of my job to occasionally deal with intimidating doctors and supervisors. I learned to let them vent, use humor, and consider timing when dealing with difficult ones. Once in a while I had a frustrating day, but who didn't?

Perhaps one of the most demoralizing and insidious problems in healthcare systems is the incidence of workplace violence.

✓ A press release issued by the American Nurses Association (February 9, 2000) states that nursing homes and hospitals hold the dubious distinction of being the sites of almost two thirds (64%) of all nonfatal workplace assaults.

Dorrie's Story continued

When I accepted a new position at an inner-city neighborhood health center, I couldn't wait to get started. It was the perfect job for me at this stage in my career. I felt confident in my nursing skills and believed I had a lot to both offer and learn in this busy clinic. I was especially excited that I would be working with a woman doctor and NP, both self-described feminists. How cool, I thought, working with women and no more big male egos to deal with. I fully expected it to feel great!

We have many definitions, labels, and excuses for a wide array of abusive behaviors in our workplaces. Horizontal or lateral and vertical violence, Interactive Work Place Trauma, (IWPT), bullying, disruptive behavior, physical and verbal, or covert and overt abuse are all terms which reflect aggressive, passive, or passive-aggressive behaviors.

Dorrie's Story continued

No matter how hard I tried to establish a collegial relationship, the physician, Martha, wasn't buying it. Day in and day out, I put up with her volatile temperament and excessive demands. Nothing I did to try to build a sense of shared accomplishment or basic trust worked. I couldn't get over the irony that this feminist physician, a potential heroine, treated me like crap. Slowly but surely, I became miserable in my job.

The International Council of Nurses (ICN) defines abuse as "behavior that humiliates, degrades, or otherwise indicates a lack of respect for the dignity and worth of an individual," (ICN, 2007).[15] The manifestations of abuse vary greatly, but they do have one thing in common, a lack of respect – for ourselves or someone else.

✓ Most surveys show 80-97 % of nurses experience verbal abuse.[16]

Aggressive behavior sits at the top of the oppression totem pole and passive behavior sits at the bottom. Lurking in between are a variety of passive-aggressive behaviors. Our voices are part of our self-expression.

---

15 *International Council of Nurses. (ICN) 2007. "Guidelines on Coping with Violence in the Workplace," retrieved from ICN website 02/09, http://www.icn.ch/guide_violence.pdf.*

16 *See Laura Sofield's website, www.laurasofield.com for researlch and articles on workplace violence.*

When we don't have the skills, opportunities, and supports for healthy expressions, we find other ways. In fact, we are pretty creative about it!

Dorrie's Story continued

One day while trying to find a patient's record, Martha stormed up to me in full view of the waiting room and yelled, "What the hell are you doing with the charts? You need to find O'Rourke's file NOW! Do you understand?" I fought back tears. It wasn't the first time this had happened, but it really got to me that day. I was so angry, but I didn't want to give in to my emotional state. I told myself to focus on the patient. I had seen the lab results come in on her biopsy, and I knew she was going to get some tough news. I took a deep breath, gritted my teeth, and said that I would "find it right away."

The physician who yells at a nurse to "get somebody in here who knows what they are doing," the nurse manager who tells a staff nurse that she should try to be less sensitive about a colleague's abrupt behavior, the staff nurse who doesn't mention to the traveling nurse that the glucose test strips she's looking for were relocated, the unit coordinator who rolls her eyes when the new nurse

> *It means a great deal to those who are oppressed to know that they are not alone. And never let anyone tell you that what you are doing is insignificant.*
>
> **--Bishop Desmond Tutu**

asks a question, and the nurse who avoids calling a physician to report a change in their patient's status are all examples of abusive behavior.[17]

Dorrie's Story continued

I went back to the front desk. Valerie, our unit coordinator, was sitting there talking with a new nurse. I could see O'Rourke's file, which made me furious. I snatched it and gave her the most piercing angry look I could muster. "Thanks a lot!" I snapped. She rolled her eyes, and I heard her mutter something to the nurse, as I hurried to get the chart to the doctor. When I dropped the chart on her desk, Martha didn't even look up.

It may seem like strong language to describe avoidant behavior or non-verbal innuendo as abuse, yet, in my opinion, when people use their power or voice in a way that disrespects someone else, it is just that.

Dorrie's Story continued

Later that day, I went to my supervisor. I was determined to do something and knew I could not take Martha's abuse any more. I told her how Martha had treated me and that it was a daily experience. I explained how frustrated I was, and that I had tried everything humanly possible to build a working relationship. My supervisor just shrugged and said, "Yeah, she's hard to work with, but she takes good care of her patients." She told me that she heard Valerie

17 Although not specific to nursing or healthcare, Patricia Evans is a pioneer in writing and speaking on verbally abusive relationships and offers many resources available via her websites, www.patriciaevans.com and www.verbalabuse.com.

complaining to the new nurse about me and wondered if I was "having trouble at home."

If we think of assertiveness as a cultural mindset, where respecting others and ourselves is the definition, we can use this model to develop an organizational goal. Speaking up and listening respectfully could be considered different learning needs for building assertiveness! The aggressive person needs training in listening, the passive person in speaking up, and the passive-aggressive individual could benefit from both! With the right training and leadership commitment, these dysfunctional relationships can be turned around.

Dorrie's Story continued Version A

I was stunned. I finally went to get some help from my supervisor, and all of a sudden I'm in trouble for mistreating Valerie. The idea that I was having trouble at home was so infuriating. What about the trouble I was having at work?

"That's it!" I told my supervisor. "I've had it. I am not doing this anymore. I know what it is like to work in an environment where I am respected and this isn't it. I'm officially giving you a two-week notice right now."

My supervisor stared at me. "I'm sorry to hear that Dorrie, but I'll let Human Resources know"

Dorrie's Story continued Version B

I tried to understand my supervisor's approach and accept the status quo. I gained weight and increasingly dreaded going into work. Three months ago, I hurt my back helping a patient get on the exam table. I went out on workers comp disability. I feel sick when I think about going back.

Dorrie's Story continued Version C

When Martha yelled at me, I told her that it was inappropriate, and I would not tolerate abusive behavior from anyone. I reported the incident to my supervisor who backed me up and also spoke with Martha. The unit was supported by a strong Human Resources policy which was enforced. I'm still working there and love my job. Martha and I have had some challenges, but we have grown from them and have developed mutual respect. I am always learning from her, and, sometimes, she learns from me.

✓ According to the findings from the 2004 National Sample Survey of Registered Nurses by the U.S. Department of Health and Human Services, an estimated 488,000 RNs with active licenses are not employed in nursing. This represents about 17 % of the total RN population.

Summary

Workplace violence is an insidious and pervasive part of our culture. Regardless of cause or intention, it leaves in its wake a destructive influence on relationships and communication. Mistrust and fear become embedded into key issues such as quality, safety, staffing, and job satisfaction. We tolerate, excuse, avoid, and cope.

> *It is no measure of health to be well adjusted to a profoundly sick society.*
>
> **--Jiddu Krishnamurti**

- ✓ He had a very stressful day.

- ✓ I'm used to it. It helps to develop a thick skin. That's what I tell the new grads.

- ✓ I reported him once and never heard anything.

- ✓ Deep inside she has a heart of gold.

- ✓ He's a great physician/nurse etc.

- ✓ I know Dr. Smith will be angry if I call this late. I'll wait and see if the patient's blood pressure drops any further.

- ✓ It is part of my job. Nothing will ever change.

Yet nevertheless, because we are human beings, this kind of culture takes its toll. We may become afraid to ask questions, give or receive feedback, request or offer help, share ideas, or admit to and learn from mistakes.

We may develop resentments and dread going into work and maybe even, covertly or overtly, spread abuse ourselves.

Creating cultures where there is a zero tolerance for abuse is paramount. The message must be consistent and clear. There is no room for double standards or mixed messages. Everyone in the organization must be accountable, including senior management and physicians.

✓ The shortage of registered nurses (RNs) in the U.S. could reach as high as 500,000 by 2025 according to a report released by Dr. Peter Buerhaus and colleagues in March 2008. The report, titled "The Future of the Nursing Workforce in the United States: Data, Trends and Implications," found that the demand for RNs is expected to grow by 2% to 3% each year.

The healthiest outcome for Dorrie, in my opinion, is the one where she speaks up to Martha right away. However, in order for this to be a realistic outcome in a facility with a history of toxic dynamics, she must have the skills to speak up appropriately, the physician and her supervisor must be better equipped to listen respectfully, and the organizational culture must clearly and consistently support all of the players in these efforts.

In the next few chapters, we will explore in more detail how individuals can improve their communication skills as well as the role organizations must play in order to promote successful outcomes.

Discussion Questions

1. Margaret J. Wheatley, quoted in this chapter, describes aggression as a nearly invisible medium common in organizations. What do you think she means by this?

2. How many examples of aggressive, passive, or passive-aggressive behaviors can you find in Dorrie's story?

3. Why do you suppose Dorrie accepted the idea that dealing with intimidating physicians and supervisors was part of her job?

4. Do you know any nurses who are not practicing? Why do you think they are not, and what ideas do you have that would encourage their return to the profession?

5. Think of one of your most rewarding experiences as a nurse and exchange stories with a colleague.

Reflection Questions

1. Which of the three different outcomes (version A, B, or C) for Dorrie's situation seem most likely to you?

2. In this chapter, I use the word abuse to include avoidant behavior and non-verbal behaviors. What are your thoughts about using of the word abuse in this way?

3. What experiences do you have with vertical and/or horizontal violence in your career as a nurse?

4. Have you ever thought of leaving the profession? What would make you stay or leave?

Part II: Building Communication Skills & Workplace Support

Overview

The middle section of this book is devoted to building assertiveness and respectful listening skills. We will also explore strategies for creating organizational cultures where these effective communication and respectful relationships can thrive. Like three legs of a stool, all of these elements must be functioning in order to create and sustain positive workplaces.

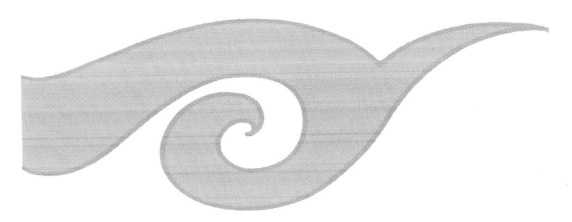

Chapter Five

Speaking Up Assertively

Assertiveness means different things to different people. Some view it as a negative attribute and believe that assertive people are pushy, dominating, or inconsiderate. Others view it more positively, as a necessary ability to stand up for yourself. Even a search in online dictionaries reveals differing definitions.

> The world is moved along, not only by the mighty shoves of its heroes, but also by the aggregate of tiny pushes of each honest worker.
>
> **--Helen Keller**

For our purposes, speaking our truth, being assertive, and speaking up are all suitable expressions for describing people who:

- ✓ Report concerns, ask questions, and give feedback confidently.

- ✓ Are aware when their rights, feelings, or opinions are being compromised.

- ✓ Respect the views of others, even when disagreeing.

- ✓ Express feelings and emotions appropriately and with ease.

- ✓ Avoid raising their voices and using disrespectful language when communicating with others.

- ✓ Say no or set other limits when they need to.

✓ Feel safe to participate in group situations (listening and speaking up).

✓ Are able to take responsibility for their thoughts and actions.

✓ Ask for what they need or want respectfully.

✓ Are able to approach conflict collaboratively.

There are many training models that help to build assertiveness. Some examples that we see in healthcare include:

✓ **SBAR** (situation, background, assessment, and recommendation) is one model currently being introduced into healthcare organizations. SBAR has its origins in the military and attempts to standardize and clarify reporting efforts where critical information is being transmitted.

✓ **The Speak Up Initiative** of The Joint Commission builds assertiveness into healthcare settings by encouraging patients to have input into their care.

✓ **Judy Ringer**, of Power & Presence Training, teaches "Purposeful Communication." By asking ourselves, before we speak, what purpose our communication intends to serve, we take responsibility for our thinking and are more likely to express ourselves respectfully and successfully. Determining the purpose for the communication supports us in speaking up assertively.

✓ **VitalSmarts®** company provides an array of resources including: Crucial Conversations® Training which teaches skills for creating alignment and agreement by fostering open dialogue around high-stakes topics. The book, *Crucial Conversations: Tools for Talking When Stakes are High*[18] has become a well-known resource connected with this organization.

I suspect that any tool used by an individual or organization can contribute to building assertiveness, and I also believe that these four models are making important contributions to addressing assertiveness issues in healthcare systems. The strategies presented in *Confident Voices* add to the foundation for any such training involving nurses for two important reasons.

> *All learning has an emotional base.*
>
> **--Plato**

First, this book combines communication and conflict expertise with insights about the underlying dynamics and nature of day-to-day nursing practice. Second, *Confident Voices* focuses on the practice and discussion of these skills among nurse professionals. In short, these strategies bring the work home! No matter how straightforward the intellectual aspects of communication skill building are, the changes in behavior required are extraordinarily challenging.

Practicing and learning assertiveness is complicated! It requires personal growth in areas of self-respect and self-esteem. In addition, nurses often work under great pressure. Every day we must stretch our perceived limitations to, and sometimes beyond, healthy maximum capacities. The environments we work in are constantly changing, with new treatments,

---

18 Crucial Conversations: Tools for Talking When Stakes are High, *Kerry Patterson, Joseph Grenny, Ron McMillan, and Al Switzler, 2002, McGraw-Hill.*

knowledge, technology, and regulations to absorb. We must provide sophisticated and compassionate care in the midst of volatile patient, family, and caregiver dynamics; a relentless barrage of call bells, lights, alarms, and phones; and constantly shifting priorities, all of which are urgent to someone! It is a tough environment in which to practice new skills, especially when they are difficult skills to learn!

"I" Statements as an Assertiveness Tool

In this chapter we will review, practice, and reflect on the use of "I" statements as a method for building assertiveness. In my teaching and training experience, I find that most people are familiar with the "I" statement format, but many are unsure how to use it in real-life situations. Because assertiveness involves self-esteem and self-esteem is often an issue for nurses, including myself, this focus on "I" statements is important. Ultimately, assertive language does not always require "I" statements per se, yet there is an inherent value of self in all assertiveness. For this reason, I strongly recommend this focus as part of assertiveness training for nurses.

I find "I" statements challenging, especially when I am feeling vulnerable. I also know from consulting with organizations and teaching professionals at a variety of levels, that many people, including senior leaders, are often amazed at how tricky using "I" statements can be!

Opportunities for guided practice are limited and yet are critical for developing the skill. One of my graduate students shared that she had tried using an "I" statement with a colleague following our classroom discussion and, "It didn't go so well." She was willing to talk about the experience and was patient with my probing for more details. She enriched everyone's learning by explaining how she had been so frustrated with a colleague's noisy behavior in the hall that she yelled at her to "Shut up." Following that, she approached the colleague with an "I" statement and made a point to include a list of irritating things that had been building into resentments for months!

Unfortunately, in this case, the "I" statement was embedded in blame and judgment, and the conflict, not surprisingly, escalated. The good news is that the student realized that her approach had some room for improvement. It would have been very easy for her to conclude that using "I" statements was dangerous and stop trying. However, the potential for healing, ownership, role modeling, and authentic relationship-building grew with this student's willingness to try, reflect, and do her own work. What a great testimony to her leadership!

There is considerable variation in describing "I" statements, and even experts may disagree about how and when they are best used. Nevertheless, they are valuable tools, because they help navigate conflict while building self-awareness and self-respect.

"I" statements are considered to be components of assertiveness when they:

- ✓ Build and nourish relationships.

- ✓ Lead to problem solving.

- ✓ Validate our own perspective and create room for others.

- ✓ Are less likely to provoke a defensive response.

✓ Can be direct and honest.

✓ Increase the chances for effective communication.

✓ Are useful tools when we are upset.

✓ Use compromise and collaboration to settle conflict.

✓ Help to build self-awareness and self-respect.

"I" statements may not be effective tools when:

✓ Used with small children.

✓ Are disguised "You" or "They" statements.

✓ You are in unsafe situations.

"I" Statement Format

You've probably come across a format for "I" statements. Here is the one I use in the workshops and classes I teach:

I feel _____ when you _____ because _____ and I would like _____ .

For example, let's say your colleagues are talking loudly at the nurses' station while you are documenting. Here are two different ways you could address the situation:

> *I'm frustrated with the volume of your discussion because I can't concentrate on my documentation. I would appreciate it if you would talk more quietly.*

OR

> *You need to quiet down. I can't document in the middle of your loud talking!*

See how the language in the first one includes ownership and asks for something, whereas the second example is blaming and demanding? On the other hand, it is perfectly reasonable to argue that the second example can be a valid option in certain circumstances.

Ultimately, the effectiveness of using "I' statements depends on the relationship as it exists now and what you would like that relationship to be in the future. If there is a basis of trust and respect in place, then even a simple, "Shhhh, I'm trying to work," would probably be OK. If there is mistrust or other underlying factors, then such a statement may very well be inflammatory.

Imagine your supervisor has been giving you more and more work above your normal duties, and now she is giving you another project. Compare these two examples of addressing the situation:

> *I'm overwhelmed with the new project you are asking me to work on because I'm already stressed by my current assignments. If you are going to give me additional work, I'll need your help in prioritizing and/or to get some additional support.*

OR

My supervisor is driving me crazy. She keeps on piling up the work and doesn't care about how it affects me. I can't do it all. I can't stand working for her.

Notice how, in the first example, there is an opportunity to set a limit respectfully with a direct conversation. In the second example, there is an attempt to build an alignment against the leader by complaining behind his/her back. How safe and skilled an employee is in taking a direct approach will again be based on the relationship that exists and the one she wants to exist. The response of the leader in this case would also contribute to the dynamics of either circumstance.

> *Leap and the net shall appear.*
>
> **--Julia Cameron**

Here are two different ways of addressing a leadership scenario in which one of your staff has been working really hard on a patient assignment that is stressful for her.

I'm concerned that this patient assignment is creating a lot of stress for you and can see that you are working really hard. Is there anything I can do or that you need to help you to manage your workload with less stress?

OR

If she needs help, she's going to have to ask for it. I don't have the time or energy to coddle her. Besides, no one offered me any help when I worked that floor.

It is pretty obvious, when viewed through our objective lens, that the former statement builds the relationship and allows the leader to become a supportive resource. If the employee asks for help that the leader is unable to provide, a new problem can surface and be dealt with. In the second example, there is no opportunity for this resolution. Issues such as time limitations or training needs may remain under the radar while hidden resentments and resistance are cultivated.

Understanding what we want in terms of our relationships is a key factor in figuring out how to achieve them.

<u>The Spirit of "I' Statements</u>

Using the "I" statement format is a great way to enhance your practice, and it can be a useful tool when you are under pressure. On the other hand, it can be awkward and may interfere with the flow of natural dialogue. For this reason, it can be helpful to gain a sense of the spirit behind "I" statements – remembering to show ownership for your role and respect for others.

Being clear about what you need and what you want will set the tone for others to do the same. This, in and of itself, can turn a potential power struggle into a collaborative process and, for this reason, can be a powerful tool for promoting positive workplaces. When combined with clear limit-setting about what you are able and willing to do, the possibilities for creative problem solving can flourish.

Ownership of the problem will typically involve some degree of risk-taking in terms of revealing yourself to others. How much you decide to share is a personal decision, which will vary greatly. Look for ways to be open without making yourself overly vulnerable.

For example:

I'm upset about your tone of voice for personal reasons.

is quite different from*:*

I'm a nervous wreck because of my history of being in an abusive relationship.

You have a right to privacy, and you may want to be cautious about what you share and with whom. It is fine to proceed slowly. You can always share more information as you develop your relationship.

Here is an "I" statement checklist that you may find helpful in practicing assertiveness. The more of these you find pertinent to your situation, the more helpful the strategy will be.

"I" Statement Checklist

✓ I am trying to repair, build, or maintain a relationship.

✓ I want to find a solution that works for both of us.

✓ I value and respect my own opinion.

✓ I value and respect the opinion of others.

✓ I am willing to disclose an appropriate amount of personal information.

✓ I am open to ideas from another.

✓ I am willing to compromise or collaborate.

✓ I am being honest.

Practice "I" Statements

You are now ready for the "I" statement challenge! Use the format, spirit, and/or checklist to come up with revisions of the following statements. Examples of effective "I" statements are found at the end of the chapter, but remember, there are lots potential variations. If your ideas are significantly different, compare your thoughts with the checklist above and /or discuss variations with a colleague.

> Our awareness is always in training. We can learn and practice new skills to change the way we handle conflict and the way we live.
>
> **--Judy Ringer**

The "I" Statement Challenge!

Turn the following statements into ones that show ownership and respect for you and the other person. Sample answers are found at the end of this chapter. Discuss them with a colleague. There are many "right" answers!

1. You make me so mad when you leave a pile of charts in the break room.

    _____

    _____

    _____

2. Dr. Jones is always mumbling about which Betadine solution she wants and then yells at me when I don't have the right one at the bedside. I hate working with her.

    _____

    _____

    _____

3. I think you are an inconsiderate, arrogant creep! How dare you call me incompetent and criticize my assessment skills in front of my colleagues?

    _____

    _____

    _____

4. She never does her share of the prep work.

_____

_____

_____

5. You are so selfish. You don't care about me one bit. All you do is spend time with your friends.

_____

_____

_____

6. You ought to get more exercise.

_____

_____

_____

7. Most people would complain about the number of times you are late.

_____

_____

_____

8. You never admit when you are wrong.

_____

_____

_____

9. You are a self-righteous, inconsiderate power-monger.

_____

_____

_____

10. The whole team is fed up with you calling out sick.

_____

_____

_____

11. Those nurses on 5 East don't know what they are talking about.

_____

_____

_____

12. It is sickening how she gets rewarded for smoking by taking more breaks than the rest of us.

_____

_____

_____

Before we leave the topic, there are some gray areas that you should be aware of.

Gray Areas Regarding "I" Statements

Using "I" statements in healthcare provider-to-patient situations requires caution for several reasons.

✓ Patients are in a dependent position. Our role requires that we provide care and expertise to help them be healthier.

✓ We must be aware of what our feelings are and where they are coming from. This means we have developed awareness about any triggers we may have and/or secondary gains we may benefit from in the dependent nurse/patient relationship.

✓ We must be able to discern what is appropriate to share with patients about our feelings and what is not. This does not mean we bury feelings, but rather find alternate resources for support. Sometimes we may be worried, annoyed, and anxious all at once!

✓ We must also be able to discern what is reasonable to ask patients to do for their health rather than for meeting our needs.

Consider these nurse-to-patient examples:

I need you to be honest with me about your chest pain. I take every complaint of chest pain very seriously.

I'm upset when you don't follow instructions and keep coming back with problems that could be prevented.

Statements with "I" frames can be effective and non-threatening ways to set limits or to encourage compliance. What we share about ourselves, and what we can expect patients to do in response to our needs, requires caution and judgment. When in doubt, run it by a colleague.

The previous examples are not necessarily bad, but I might amend both:

I need you to be honest with me about your chest pain. I take every complaint of chest pain very seriously. As your nurse professional, I want to make sure that you are getting the treatment you need. Your description of symptoms is critical information and will help us to make the best recommendations.

I'm feeling a little frustrated when you keep coming back to the clinic with problems that could be prevented. I want to help you understand how to prevent problems, yet I don't seem to be helping you. What thoughts do you have about this? Do you have any ideas that would help us both be more successful?

There may be some patients for whom these statements would be appropriate and some for whom they are not. You must consider each case separately. In fine-tuning this work, ask yourself the following questions:

> *Is it fair for me to ask the patient to do this for me? Or is it more appropriate for me to express my concerns to a team member?*

With courage you will dare to take risks, have the strength to be compassionate, and the wisdom to be humble. Courage is the foundation of integrity.

-- Keshavan Nair

Using "I" statements in leadership roles is also tricky, yet it can be done by keeping the following in mind:

✓ What is appropriate to share with staff about your feelings?

✓ Being clear about limits, expectations, and consequences and acting on them consistently may be more appropriate than asking an employee to do something differently. In other words, if an employee on your unit is repeatedly late, make sure she understands that being on time is expected and that continued tardiness will result in disciplinary action. Then follow through. You can offer resources to help the individual, such as an employee assistance program, and express your concern for her job and personal health, but keep these separate from the expectations and consequences.

Consider this example:

> *I'm frustrated when you come into work late on a regular basis. I expect you to be on time. Please let me know if there is some way I can help you be successful with this. This is a performance issue, and it is my job to hold you accountable.*

Take another look at the examples in the "I" statement challenge and see how you might revise them if you were in a leadership position.

"You", "She/he" or "They" Statements

It is not unusual for many of us get caught up in blaming and/or defending ourselves rather than owning our part of a conflict or problem. Rather than framing an issue from our own perspective, it is easier or safer to point out what someone else is doing. The language we use shows up in many of the challenging statements mentioned previously.

"You", "She/he" or "They" statements undermine assertiveness when they:

✓ Avoid responsibility for our feelings.

✓ Blame and/or judge others.

✓ Present opinions as if they were facts.

✓ Don't allow room for other perspectives.

✓ Are often authoritarian, controlling, or "put-downs."

✓ Can provoke defensiveness and/or resistance in others.

✓ Tend to keep the conflict going.

✓ Are a form of manipulation.

✓ Are sweeping generalizations.

It can be a fun and eye-opening activity to spend a day simply noticing when such statements come up in conversations. As you notice them, simply wonder whether there might be room for more ownership.

Disguised "I" Statements

In addition to language variations, personal options, and gray areas, "I" statements can also be disguised "You" statements. Consider these comments:

I feel like you have never cared about me and never will.

I feel like you are an ignorant, arrogant creep.

Both of the above comments start out with "I feel," but neither shows ownership or mutual respect. It is easy to fall into this trap when we haven't practiced the skill enough or are especially angry, hurt, or vulnerable. Disguised comments such as these can be confusing, abusive, and unfortunately give the practice of "I" statements a bad reputation.

"I" Statement Challenge Answers

Here are some examples of appropriate revisions that I have come up with. Keep in mind that there are many variations depending on circumstances, relationships, and other preferences. If you find one that is particularly challenging or that you disagree with, don't forget to run it by a colleague. If you are still wondering about it, feel free to send me an email outlining your thoughts. Put *Confident Voices* in the subject field and I will do my best to get back to you. (bbbboynton@earthlink.net).

1. **You make me so mad when you leave a pile of charts in the break room.**

   I get upset when I see you leave a pile of charts in the break room. It is not an appropriate place to leave them, and I worry about confidentiality and wasting time looking for charts I need. I'd appreciate it if you would document or review charts in the appropriate area.

2. **Dr. Jones is always mumbling about which Betadine solution she wants and then yells at me when I don't have the right one at the bedside. I hate working with her.**

   Dr. Jones, I can't understand what you are saying. We have 5 Betadine solutions on the unit. Which one do you want for the debridement that I am going to assist you with on our patient?

3. **I think you are an inconsiderate, arrogant creep! How dare you call me incompetent and criticize my assessment skills in front of my colleagues?**

   I'm angry because of the way you criticized me in front of my colleagues. I felt humiliated by your language and tone. Please find ways to share your knowledge without name-calling in public.

4. **She never does her share of the prep work.**

   I feel overwhelmed with the amount of prep work I have to do and would like to talk about a way to distribute the work so that I can do a good job in a reasonable time frame.

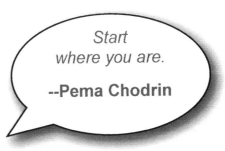

Start where you are.

--Pema Chodrin

5. **You are so selfish. You don't care about me one bit. All you do is spend time with your friends.**

   I feel hurt when you spend so much time with your friends, because I feel like I am not a priority to you. I'd like to figure a way to spend more time together.

6. **You ought to get more exercise.**

   I feel sad when I see you watching TV all day because I worry that you are not getting enough exercise. You are a very important person in my life, and I want you to be around for a long time. Would you please consider taking better care of yourself? Is there any way I could help?

7. **Most people would complain about the number of times you are late.**

   I'm frustrated with your coming in late to work. This is the third time this week, and I can't get out on time when you are not available for report. I need to trust that you will be on time and will talk with our supervisor if this continues.

8. **You never admit when you are wrong.**

   I feel frustrated when you blame me for every problem we have. I am willing to look at my contribution and would appreciate it if you would take ownership of your part.

9. **You are a self-righteous, inconsiderate power-monger.**

   I'm confused with the way you have organized this project. My ideas and concerns never seem to be validated or used. I'd appreciate the opportunity to be a more active participant in this project.

10. **The whole team is fed up with you calling out sick.**

    I'm getting exasperated with the number of sick calls you've been making. I'm finding it difficult to depend on you and am worried about resentments that I, and possibly others, are feeling. I'm sorry that you are having health problems and would like to make some time to hear about what's going on for you and learn if there is any thing I can do to help. Would you be willing to talk about this?

11. **Those nurses on 5 East don't know what they are talking about.**

    I'm concerned about the number of readmits we are getting from 5E discharges. I wonder how we could find out more about them and address any training or other needs that arise.

12. It is sickening how she gets rewarded for smoking by taking more breaks than the rest of us.

I feel taken advantage of when you take more breaks than I do. I'd like to have equal opportunities to get off the floor for a few minutes during the day. What ideas do you have for making sure that we are taking breaks evenly?

Summary

"I" statements are far more complicated than they appear to be on the surface. They can be messy and gray with lots of "right" ways to compose them. Nevertheless, they are an integral part of assertive language and contribute greatly to collaborative cultures. The more we can integrate ownership and respect into our workplace communication, the healthier our relationships will be!

Interdependency follows independence.

--Stephen Covey

Discussion Questions

1. Review the list of expressions that describe people who are assertive, speak their truth, and speak up assertively with a colleague. Do you think these are important in healthcare settings? What is your reasoning?

2. Choose two or three samples answers from the "I" statement activity and write down alternative phrasing that meets the criteria for the spirit of "I" statements. How could these statements be different for a relationship that is secure versus one that is strained?

3. Choose two or three sample answers from the "I" statement activity, discuss how the listener might feel, and then respond to both the example and the revision.

4. Consider the interdependence of speaking up, listening, and safe cultures. What might happen to others when one or two aren't functioning in a healthy way?

Reflection Questions

1. How does the word assertiveness come across to you?

2. What kinds of stressors have you experienced in your career?

3. Have you ever had an "I" statement backfire? Is there anything you would do differently given insights from this chapter?

4. Can you think of any examples where you might apply differing approaches in order to build or maintain a work relationship?

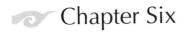 Chapter Six

Respectful Listening

Communication in its simplest state includes three components: sender, message, and receiver. Individuals and organizations wishing to maximize communication will be more effective if they seek ways to allocate responsibility to recipients of the information as well as to the senders. When other barriers are present, such as verbal abuse, stress, and/ or intimidating power differences, respectful listening must be part of the landscape.

> *I know that you believe you understand what you think I said, but I'm not sure you realize that what you heard is not what I meant.*
>
> **-- Robert McCloskey**

Consider the ramifications when individuals in any team are taught and expected to speak up without putting the same effort into teaching them to listen to what is being said. How far can strategies geared to speaking up go if we are not paying attention to what's being said and how it is being received? We commonly think of assertiveness as a process of expression, yet we may have much to gain by considering it a mindset. An assertive mindset creates room for respecting and developing skills associated with listening and speaking up.

Respectful Listening

Respectful listening doesn't necessarily involve agreeing with, or making changes because of, what someone else says. In its most basic form, respectful listening is a process for understanding someone else. It is a powerful gift and, when used effectively, involves learning about another person's perspective which may include his/her thoughts, observations, ideas, or experience. We may even learn surprising information about how someone perceives what we are saying. If this is different from our intention, we can try a different approach. If we are open, we can gain insight about how our communication style might influence others and keep this in mind for future conversations.

> *We do not believe in ourselves until someone reveals that deep inside us something is valuable, worth listening to, worthy of trust, sacred to our touch. Once we believe in ourselves we can risk curiosity, wonder, spontaneous delight or any experience that reveals the human spirit.*
>
> **--E.E. Cummings**

Our ability to separate listening and learning from our own responses can be extraordinarily challenging. Intellectually, we know what respectful listening is, but emotionally, it can be quite difficult to practice. When we are able to keep our own reactions and opinions out of the listening process, we will be more successful at clarifying and validating another's perspective. Along with "I" statements, this is an effective tool for diffusing a power struggle and engaging others in a collaborative effort.

Again, respectful listening is not so much an intellectual challenge as it is an emotional one. I believe we all know what effective listening is supposed to be, but don't always have opportunities to build and practice this important skill. Here is a review of the essential ingredients for respectful listening.

Maximize Openness to Other Perspectives

Listening respectfully involves being open to another's viewpoint. It is especially challenging when another person's perspective includes an opposing opinion. This openness to other points of view does not mean giving up your own opinion or even changing it.

You need to be willing to understand where someone else is coming from as a totally separate experience from where you are coming from. This is easier said than done. We can use these common optical illusions from the public domain to help emphasize this point.

<u>Perspective-taking Challenge</u>

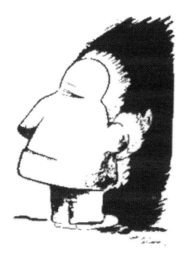

In the image above, briefly describe what you see in the box. Most likely, some of you will see one image and some of you will see two. When I first looked at this, I saw a man's head, facing left with eyes closed. If this is what you see, your perspective is similar to mine. Others of you will initially see a person with a winter coat going into a cave or perhaps an eskimo going into an igloo. As a simple optical illusion, it can be fun to test our visual observations and compare to others.

There is also a deep learning opportunity about perspective here. If you saw both perspectives in the first example, you will appreciate the learning in one or both of the next two examples. If you saw only one, you can take a moment now and think about what helped you to see a different perspective. Were you able to see the alternate one when I described it? What happened to your perspective when you were able to see a new one? The ability to see different points of view is a critical listening skill.

Try following similar steps for the next image without my cues. Can a colleague, friend, or family member help to show you a point of view that you would have missed? Can you help another person to see two different images?

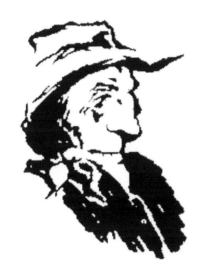

_____

_____

Now let's build on this idea with this slightly different activity. Consider the drawing below and ask yourself to describe what it could be. Ask a colleague what ideas he/she has. There are no wrong answers. They are just different ways of looking at the same thing.

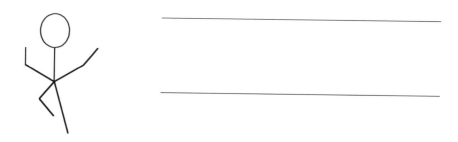

<u>Stay In the Present</u>

Any tool that keeps you focused on a verbal exchange will help create the space needed to take in what someone else is saying. Often, while we are supposedly listening, the need to defend our position or our need to plan for the future is unfolding in our mind. It is a natural human response, yet is counterproductive with respect to listening. Working to minimize the "internal buzz"

> *We encourage others to change only if we honor who they are now."*
>
> **--Margaret J. Wheatley and Myron Kellner- Roger**

will save time in the long run, because it will help you come to a mutual understanding the first time around.

There are a variety of meditations, prayers, and breathing exercises, that can help you stay calm or regain calmness when you are stressed. My friend and colleague, Judy Ringer, author of *Unlikely Teachers: Finding the Hidden Gifts in Daily Conflict,*[19] teaches a process called "Centering" from the martial art, aikido. I have found her to be a wonderful teacher and asked her to write about a centered approach to listening for this book. She shares the following with us:

---

19 *Ringer, Judy, Unlikely Teachers: Finding the Hidden Gifts in Daily Conflict, 2006, One Point Press, Portsmouth, NH, 2006. Also see www.judyringer.com.*

Centered Response to Listening from Judy Ringer

Centering yourself can be as simple as taking a breath. We've all heard and perhaps spoken the word many times, but we usually do not associate centering with a mind-body quality that includes increased awareness as well as physical stability. When we're centered, we become more present to our surroundings, and therefore more capable of managing whatever comes our way, verbally and non-verbally.

In aikido, we use a physical centering practice that allows us to feel the quality of center in our bodies. Our physical center of gravity is approximately two inches below the navel. In aikido, we call it tanden, or one-point. When I focus on the body's center, I become more balanced in all ways. Breathing from center, I more easily manage my own thoughts and emotions, and I access the still, calm origin of my ki (my energy or life force).

There is a simple exercise you can do with a partner that demonstrates the power of the centered state:

1. Without being centered, ask someone to push on you with a gentle and steady pressure. You can choose any spot you like, though I usually use the sternum or the middle of the upper back.

2. Notice what happens. Do you wobble? Do you resist by pushing your body against the pressure?

3. Now center yourself. Bring your awareness to the tanden. Breathe in and out a few times.

4. As you exhale, ask your partner to push again in the same way, this time mentally redirecting the push energy toward and through your tanden into the floor. Instead of pushing back or feeling pushed, bring the energy of your partner's hand to you and imagine the push as energy you can engage and use.

5. Notice what happens. Were you more stable? How did you engage and redirect the energy?

6. Once you have practiced this physical centering process, notice that you feel stable in other ways–emotionally, mentally, and spiritually. Understand that with practice, you can do this anytime and all by yourself.

7. It is an easy next step to center yourself while listening. Recalling how you managed the push of your centering partner's hand, you can use the eye contact, words, gestures, even the physical proximity of the speaker in a similar way. Centering will help you quiet your internal dialogue and be perfectly present, even when the speaker communicates ideas you may not agree with. When you're centered, you can be patient and listen with your whole body.

Use Receptive Body Language, Tone, and Non-verbal Communication

Up to 93% of our communication takes place in the non-verbal zone. This means that our facial expressions, physical stance, and tone of voice are all conveying powerful messages. Dealing with conflict face-to-face will almost always lead to a much richer exchange, because there is so much more information being transmitted and received. Although sometimes a benefit, there can be a monumental loss of non-verbal communication when talking via email, letters, and even on the phone.

We can be mindful of receptive non-verbal communication when we are listening. Leaning in, nodding, and relaxed poses are examples of body language that shows interest and concern. Occasionally adding a "Hmmmm" or other sympathetic sound can further demonstrate that you are focused on what someone is saying.

When our words say one thing but our non-verbal communication says another, we are sending out a mixed message. Beware of mixed messages. They are often a root cause of broken trust, which is very hard to repair.

It is important to realize that body language does not always convey the language we intend. A common example is someone who is folding her arms across her chest being perceived as making a statement of resistance. I often ask workshop participants to come up with other explanations for this. I enjoy hearing their creative ideas such as: she's covering up a stain, is cold, or has a sore arm and is holding it up with the other one! (If you perceive someone as being resistant in this way, it is a great opportunity to use an "I" statement that could lead to new understanding and important feedback).

Develop True Curiosity

True curiosity is an important foundation for listening respectfully. We may use questions or strategies, such as reflecting or paraphrasing, to portray our attentiveness and to gauge our understanding. However, true curiosity comes from a deeper place and involves much more than simply asking questions. True curiosity means cultivating a sense of wonder and interest in learning more about someone else's experience. It is a tricky concept at times, because the same question may arise from true curiosity or have an agenda attached to it.

For instance, I may ask you a question about your art class because I'm curious to learn more about you, or I may be looking for a ride to the garage next to the studio where my car is being repaired.

Another example would be my asking your opinion of the new shift supervisor because I had a bad experience with her and want to tell you about it, rather than because I'm wondering about your impression. I may even want to get you on my side of a conflict.

As nurses, we are taught to use inviting language such as, "tell me more," or to ask open-ended questions when inquiring about a patient's history. Consider how much of this is a technique for obtaining accurate reports and making assessments while minimizing judgments, which may be perceived in the question.

There is nothing wrong with this. In fact, it is a therapeutic way of interacting with patients. However, sometimes there is a subtle difference between this kind of asking and true curiosity, which is not attached to anything other than an interest in understanding. Appreciating this difference can help us to cultivate pure curiosity with our workplace relationships. It is also a powerful mindset for conflict and a worthy challenge for many of us to aspire to when upset by someone else's behavior!

Open-ended questions and invitations for more information are great ways to demonstrate curiosity. Being centered, present, and working to set aside our own issues is the higher plane of true curiosity. Personally, I know that it is unrealistic to operate from this place all the time, but every once in a while I get there and when I don't, I know I'm trying.

Validate

As many of my graduate students will no doubt attest, I am a stickler for this step. In fact, for the online component of my courses in organizational conflict and communication, I have developed a validation protocol that students must use in discussing controversial healthcare topics. In a nutshell, I require that they validate their dialogue partner's opinion and receive confirmation before they are allowed to say anything about their own thinking. I do this to emphasize the idea that validating someone else's opinion is a totally separate experience from adding your own thoughts to the conversation.

In my work with leaders, I am often in a position to coach around this issue. It is not unusual for managers to be very frustrated with staff about an organizational limitation over which they have no power. Chronic power struggles and frustrations that persist between a leader and staff because of limited resources can be shifted into a collaborative mode with a fairly simple effort by the manager to validate the staff's frustration. Sometimes, it is amazing to observe or experience this shift.

For example, an executive director of a small non-profit organization was repeatedly facing the same problem with her small group of front desk staff. These three people shared the responsibility of answering the phone and greeting patients, along with other administrative duties. Unlike the rest of the staff, who had some flexible scheduling options, one of these administrative folks had to be at the desk at all times.

One day, the director decided to try the concept of validation and, instead of defending her reasons for not being able to meet the staff's request for weekly time off together, she simply said, "You sound upset about the scheduling expectation I have for you. I can see why it doesn't feel fair, and I understand your frustration at not being able to have some time off together on a regular basis."

When she told me about it later, she shared that the three women changed their facial expression and body language almost immediately. She did not go into the reasons for her decision, but made a point of asking them if she understood where they were coming from. They had been heard, and they felt it. Other possibilities for creative problem solving may have evolved once they got out of their power struggle!

Be Honest about Limitations

I have come to believe that being honest about our limitations is an almost magical prescription for evolution! When we are honest about any personal or organizational limits that may make us unavailable to someone, we show respect for ourselves and others, identify hidden or lacking resources, build trust, and create new and collaborative opportunities! As we develop our ability to listen respectfully, we automatically increase our awareness of the personal mindset and organizational resources that we need in order to practice it.

Personally, we may be preoccupied by our own life's challenges, such as family struggles, financial concerns, physical problems, or a host of other worries. Finding the emotional energy to listen to each other may or may not be realistic at any given moment.

> *I'd really like to stop and listen to you right now, but I know that I won't be able to concentrate because I'm not feeling well, (late for a meeting with my supervisor, expecting a call from my mother's doctor, having trouble with a patient's blood transfusion). I want to hear what you have to say. Can we schedule some time in the next couple of days?*

Consider how the above statement allows the other person to evaluate his/her ability to wait or perhaps seek support from someone else. Often we are so programmed to help that we may feel inadequate if we say no to someone. However, having limitations is a human reality, and it is very much OK to take care of ourselves. If we are frequently unavailable, this may shed light on a tendency to overextend, a reluctance to get support, or simply a rough patch in life.

Individually we may have a host of other priorities we are juggling or are worried about and organizationally, resources such as time, training, and private space may or may not be available to support respectful listening practices. It is probably unrealistic to think that all resources will be available at all times, and yet chronic lack of resources may be contributing to other problems.

Getting organizations to recognize the need for these supportive resources will not be easy, especially given the

> *You really can change the world if you care enough.*
>
> **-- Marion Wright Edelman**

economic and staffing issues we face. However, with more confident voices speaking up, we will connect the links between resources, staffing, and safety. In the short term, the costs of delivering healthcare may increase, but with improved safety and staffing, we are likely to see increased job and patient satisfaction. With these come decreased litigation and staff turnover, both of which are extraordinarily costly.

Recently, an MD friend of mine and I were discussing an Institute of Medicine, (IOM) report[20] which cited the direct costs of medication errors: 3.5 billion dollars per year! I passionately said to my colleague, "We have to listen more effectively!"

"We don't have time," she responded, and we both sighed. All too true perhaps, yet in my opinion, this lack of time to listen is a hidden and insidious problem that we can and must work to change.

Being clear, kind, and honest about personal and organizational limits will help these and other issues surface more effectively. With confident

---

20 Copies of Preventing Medication Errors are available from the National Academies Press, 500 Fifth Street,N.W., Lockbox 285, Washington, DC 20055; (800) 624-6242 or (202) 334-3313 (in the Washington metropolitan area); Internet, http://www.nap.edu. The full text of this report is available at http://www.nap.edu.

voices and respectful listening, issues such as workload, limited time, fatigue, and conflicting priorities will be addressed more effectively. We will increase opportunities and pressures to fix them and decrease opportunities to dismiss or delay problem-solving by attributing concerns to whining, negativity, or chronic complaining.

This is a long-term and powerful vision to absorb. Surely, one supervisor who doesn't have time or availability to listen to one staff nurse may go unnoticed, but the power of confident voices expressing limitations every day will become a visible and responsible force for change.

Practice

Respectful listening is not easy. Be patient with yourself and keep working at it. Some situations are easier than others, and there are many variables that contribute to the outcomes. Give yourself lots of credit for working at it and some slack when you need it. For me, it is harder if I am feeling rushed, stressed, or vulnerable and easier when I am relaxed, safe, and secure. I'm getting better at it, but am far from perfect, and I'm OK with that.

The Listening Challenge

This activity will help you develop your listening skills as well as your awareness about the complexities involved. Ironically, you need only listen to yourself in order to complete this challenge.

1. The first step requires you to think of an issue about which you have an opinion. A strong opinion is likely to evoke more emotional energy in the activity, but you can decide how much

risk you want to take. Your opinion can be related to nursing practice or healthcare, but it is not necessary. Also keep in mind that this is your private work. Some controversial topics include unions, abortion, and mandatory overtime. What is most important is that you have an opinion about the topic.

2. Briefly describe your opinion about the issue and why it feels important to you. Try incorporating "I" statements when you can.

3. Now try to set your perspective aside and write a brief description of an opposing or alternate view and include some reasoning that might explain why it might be important to someone else.

4. What kinds of thoughts and/or feelings does this alternative perspective bring up for you? Can you see it as a separate perspective that can exist without threatening yours?

5. How would you evaluate your ability to stay in the present? Notice if any concerns about past events or worries about anticipated repercussions are interfering with your ability to stay focused.

6. Try writing a sentence that validates the opposing opinion. You can do this by restating the opinion in a different way. If you were talking with someone, you could start such a validation by saying something like, *Let me see if I understand you correctly.*

7. What kind of body language or non-verbal communication do you think you might be prone to if you were listening to someone

express the other opinion? Do you feel like you could demonstrate more receptivity? If so, how?

8. Write down two or three questions you might ask that would show curiosity about the other opinion?

9. Can you imagine any limitations you might have regarding listening to this other viewpoint? Keep in mind that even your own feelings about the topic may make it difficult. This isn't about what you should or should not be able to do, but rather acknowledging a true limit. Something like, *I'm having a really hard time listening to your opinion, because of my own strong reaction. I'm sorry that I'm not able to listen more effectively right now. I'm going to try to get calmer. Can we try this again later?*

10. How can you reward yourself for putting some of your valuable time and energy this activity?

Summary of Respectful Listening Strategies

1. Maximize openness to other perspectives

- Remember that seeing another point of view can add to your understanding.

- You do not have to change your perspective.

2. Stay in the present

- Practice "centering" or any technique that helps you to stay calm and focused.

3. Use receptive non-verbal communication

- Roughly 80-90% of communication takes place here.

- When aligned with intent and words, this can build trust.

- When not aligned with intent and words, it can become a source of mixed messages and broken trust.

- Can be misunderstood.

4. Demonstrate true curiosity

- Think about the situation as an opportunity to learn.

- Try to set aside your own agenda or issues.

- Ask questions to seek better understanding.

- Clarify, paraphrase, and reflect what the speaker is saying.

5. Validate

- Show the speaker that you are listening and understand what s/he is saying.

- Strive to make this a separate phase of the communication.

- Value the other person.

6. Be honest about limitations

- If it is not a good time or place for you, let the person know and suggest an alternative.

- Work to minimize distractions and interruptions and, when they are unavoidable, acknowledge their impact on your ability to listen.

7. Practice

- Accept that developing great listening skills is an ongoing process and some situations are harder than others.

- Setting an example by role-modeling every chance you get.

- Give yourself credit. This is hard work!

GRRRR Model for Great Listening

Sometimes it can be helpful to have a model to use for respectful listening. I developed the GRRRR model a couple of years ago in an effort to provide a recipient-focused process for more respectful communication. It was around the time that The Joint Commission announced their requirement for structured communication, and I felt that strategies, such as SBAR and Speak Up, mentioned earlier, were not adequately addressing accountability for listeners. I believe that this is an integral part of healthcare communication problems and offer it as a simple way for organizations to ensure that both sides of the communication problem are addressed when developing structured communication protocols.

It can also be helpful to have a procedure to follow. I developed the GRRRR model with this in mind. It provides a listening protocol and can balance initiatives such as SBAR, which address the assertiveness part of structured communication. Please feel free to use this and modify it within your unit.

Greeting: Recipients can set the tone for a professional dialogue with a kind "Hello" and use of the caller's name. *Hi Beth, this is Nursing Supervisor Jones or Dr. Smith, how can I help?* This is a simple, quick, and respectful way to begin a stressful conversation.

Respectful listening: Allow clinicians to finish sentences without interruptions, with occasional acknowledgments such as, "Okay" or 'Hmmmm." A brief pause between pieces of information can decrease anxiety and allow the reporting professional an opportunity to think and transmit critical information. If the communication takes place in person, eye contact and nodding with receptive body language can promote a calm rapport, even in the middle of an emergency. When a supervisor or physician is receiving a hand-off from a clinician with lesser power, it may be helpful to realize that there may be some anxiety about bringing a concern up the ladder. Yet, this is exactly what clinicians are supposed to do.

Review: A quick summary of the information can clarify the reporter's concerns and allow for additional thoughts without being intimidating or humiliating. In addition to getting the message straight, there is enormous value in validating. A few seconds here can lead to clinicians feeling heard, respected, and ultimately understood. A challenging process, it requires the listener to separate his/her perspective and response from the clinician's report. The ability to do this can be influenced by an array of variables such as time, stress, tradition, skill, training, mood, and even the weather! Doesn't it seem prudent to establish an organizational norm rather than try to control all of these variables?

Recommend or request more information: At this stage in the communication, the responder has enough information to initiate an order or ask for more information. This will enlist and engender a team approach to problem solving. This may involve agreeing or disagreeing with the clinician's recommendation. Listeners should avoid put-downs. *A chest tube is a reasonable suggestion, and the objective information you've provided is great. This patient has some CHF too, and that could be part of the problem. Let's do a CXR and ABGs stat. Take a minute and get those tests ordered, then let's review her med list.* Leaders have opportunities here to teach and build relationships. As they do this, they can steer away from difficult dynamics and shift towards collaboration.

Reward: Positive responses such as: *Thank you for your attention to this patient's needs, I appreciate your call, or Call me if problems persist,* can help the reporter feel like a respected team player. Inviting further discussion, if needed, is an empowering leadership strategy. It reduces any reluctance to call if there are problems and simultaneously contributes to a collaborative environment.

Summary

As you can see, respectful listening requires much more of us than is obvious from an intellectual standpoint. Truly, it is a complicated and difficult process, especially in the hectic and stressful work environments in which many nurses practice. There are all sorts of strategies that each of us can work on personally and professionally. There are also many rewards – for ourselves, our colleagues, and our patients.

As we become more adept at identifying, expressing, and listening to each other's needs and limits, we will help to paint an honest picture of organizational issues that may be affecting us.

Staff RN: *I need your help in problem-solving right away.*

Supervisor: *Can it wait? I've got to go to a management meeting in 5 minutes.*

Staff RN: *No. I need your input now. I need at least 30 minutes of uninterrupted time to safely set up a stat blood transfusion for Mr. Russell, and Mrs. Jones' PCA line is infiltrated. She's complaining of pain. Can you find someone to take care of Mrs. Jones while I attend to the blood transfusion?*

Supervisor: *OK. I'll see if anyone from the ED or ICU can come up and fix the IV. If not, I'll take care of it myself.*

In this scenario both professionals are working at respectful communication and the patients are both likely to receive the care they need. If the supervisor is unable to make her management meeting and clearly expresses the reason to her supervisor, (and her supervisor listens), then the reality of staffing needs and issues will become more obvious. If this supervisor repeatedly misses management meetings for similar reasons, then the organization has the opportunity to look into this problem. Meanwhile, the staff nurse is heard and gets the support she needs to provide quality care. She also gets the message that her limits are respected and that the ultimate goal is quality care for both patients. I sometimes wonder how the evolution of unions in our profession would be different if respectful listening was a top management strategy.

As my friend and colleague, William Owens, PhD, says, "Effective listening is sometimes simple and sometimes complex, but it is always essential." It is more likely that an assertive culture will thrive when the listening aspects of communication are emphasized and attention is devoted to its importance. And, from this newly created culture of communication and respect, safer, higher quality, and more creative healthcare systems can emerge.

In the next chapter, we will take a look at the role organizations can play in building and maintaining positive workplaces for nurses.

Discussion Questions

1. Why are effective listening skills important in healthcare?

2. What are some challenges that make effective listening difficult in healthcare workplaces?

3. What ideas do you have for creating workplaces where speaking up assertively and effective listening are standard operating procedures?

Reflection Questions

1. What do you believe is your strongest listening skill? How does this contribute to creating positive workplaces?

2. Describe an opportunity where you can utilize this strength more in your professional arena?

3. From the Seven Tips on Improving Listening, choose one that you would like to work on?

4. Briefly describe a current situation at work where you feel you could practice this focus.

Chapter Seven

Creating a Safe Environment

In my classes on leadership and organizational behavior, I ask my students to think in depth about how the workplace culture impacts individuals and vice versa. For instance, what happens when you put an assertive person in an environment where passive and/or aggressive behaviors

> *Man must evolve for all human conflict a method which rejects revenge, aggression, and retaliation. The foundation of such a method is love.*
>
> **--Martin Luther King, Jr.**

are tolerated? If assertiveness means that everyone's needs are respected, then without reciprocation, it is pretty tough to maintain!

In this chapter, we will explore opportunities and reasoning for leaders to impact the organizational culture. If you are in a formal leadership position, this will give you some solid ideas for building a safe environment. In addition, it will highlight the value of leadership's role in influencing workplace dynamics. This can be of benefit whether you are a mentor, future leader, or hold an informal leadership position within your team.

Beth's Story

> When I began my consulting work several years ago, I was still working as a per diem home health nurse. I had a graduate degree in organization and management and over

*20 years of professional work as an RN, including many
years in home and occupational health positions. I had done
a lot of personal work on relationship building, boundaries,
and self-esteem. Although many growth opportunities
remain, I had, by then, gained a pretty good sense of how to
express and take of myself in healthy ways.*

Applying communication skills requires individual commitment and courage. Asking for help, owning mistakes, setting limits, and giving and receiving feedback are challenging practices and, for many of us, part of a lifetime of growth. Each time a nurse makes an effort to utilize these skills, s/he is helping build an organizational culture where healthy interactions and learning are ongoing.

But the impact on individuals alone will be limited unless the organization is also committed to change. All of the hard work that any professional does in developing respectful communication skills can be easily compromised if leadership is not genuinely invested in promoting, supporting, and enforcing the same. Change in this direction will be quicker and easier if the organization sets clear and consistent expectations for interpersonal behavior. This means that nursing, medical, and administrative leadership are all dedicated to creating and following a standard of respectful communication that applies to everyone.

Beth's Story continued

*One particular weekend, I had two situations that left me
feeling defeated and angry. First, a patient just home
following a hip replacement had shown signs of a thrombus.
I called the surgeon who angrily told me that I should call the*

PCP because it was a medical problem. I called the PCP who yelled at me because I should have called the surgeon. When I told the patient that the PCP had advised him to go to the emergency room for an evaluation, the patient yelled at me and accused me of not knowing what I was talking about. He then insisted on calling the PCP himself.

In a safe environment, everyone will be encouraged and expected to voice ideas, limits, and concerns and listen to those of others. An organization can take powerful steps towards a standard of communication that transcends differences in personality, status, generation, culture, gender, and experience.

Beth's Story continued

Although inwardly I was seething, outwardly I calmly waited while my patient called the PCP to affirm what I had already told him. I still had a long list of patients to see, and the clock was ticking. Late that Saturday night, he was admitted to the hospital and began treatment for a blood clot. The following Monday morning I was finishing paperwork and technically off duty when my supervisor came out and wanted to know why I hadn't set up the Lovenox injections to begin that day, as this patient had been discharged early that morning. I had done a great job, was exhausted from a busy weekend, and the only feedback I got was a poorly framed question that felt like an accusation.

The timing is right for this work in healthcare, and there is momentum. All of the issues we are talking about are making their way into mainstream and healthcare news. Quality and safety are hot consumer issues, as are financial concerns for healthcare businesses.

- ✓ In October of 2008, Medicare began its new practice of refusing to pay for certain "reasonably preventable" conditions such as incompatible blood transfusions, serious bed sores, and injuries from falls.

- ✓ In May of 2008, an American Nurse Association poll[21] of over 10,000 nurses nationwide revealed that 73% of nurses don't believe the staffing on their unit or shift is sufficient.

- ✓ The Institute for Healthcare Improvement is concluding **The 5 Million Lives Campaign** that was a voluntary initiative to protect patients from five million incidents of medical harm over the next two years (December 2006 – December 2008).

- ✓ The Joint Commission recently created a Sentinel Event Alert, which requires accredited organizations to develop a protocol to address intimidating and disruptive behaviors that goes into effect in January 2009.

Beth's Story continued

Another patient I went to see that day became verbally abusive when I called the doctor to discuss the cream he was using on his legs. (It was not the antibiotic one ordered on

---

21 *To view more results of ANA's Staffing Poll, or to learn more about the issue of safe staffing please visit www.safestaffingsaveslives.org/results.*

the most recent discharge paperwork.) An occupational therapist who was present tried to help by telling the patient that I was doing my job. The patient basically yelled at me to "get out." On my way out, I talked with his wife and asked if she felt safe. She assured me that she did and that it was not unusual for her husband to yell at home health staff.

Changing patients' behaviors is more complicated, because of possible mental health and/or metabolic problems, and will require additional staffing, security measures, and safety policies. This is equally important work and will be easier to address as we become clear about what abusive behaviors are and build workplaces that absolutely do not tolerate them.

Beth's Story continued

I went back to the office right away, because I was concerned that this patient might need some psychiatric intervention and wanted to contact the physician without the patient present. I ran into a colleague in the parking lot who asked me how it had gone with this patient. She told me that she had turned down this visit when she heard the scheduler say that they needed someone with a "strong personality." There was no indication of behavioral issues on the chart or scheduling board. I went to the scheduler and told her how difficult the visit was, and that I felt I should have known about the patient's behavioral issues. She said to me, "You should have asked." Shortly thereafter, the doctor yelled at me on the phone for leaving him with a

*liability issue if the client wouldn't allow or follow through on
a psychiatric evaluation.*

Any time a physician yells at a nurse, a supervisor minimizes a staff
nurse's concern, a staff nurse rolls her eyes at a nurse's aide, a manager
dismisses a complaint of bullying, or a CEO yells at an administrative
assistant, they are role modeling and perpetuating inappropriate behavior.
Recently (July 2008), a young nurse
finishing her first year of med-surg
work shared, as if it were some
sort of triumph, that she was
"finally getting used to being
yelled at." This is an alarming
statement that underscores the
need for leaders to be visible
and powerful proponents of
change.

> *Without
> aggression, it becomes
> possible to think well, to be
> curious about differences, and to
> enjoy each other's company.*
>
> **--Margaret J. Wheatley**

Beth's Story continued

*Although these were not the first instances of abusive
treatment in my career, at this stage in my life I was more
able to assess how harmful they were and how they made
me feel. I promised myself that I was not going to work in
this kind of environment anymore and left several months
later.*

Disrespectful behavior cannot be excused at any level. As we work to
change this insidious and tragic status quo, we can make room for

mistakes and forgiveness provided there is genuine, consistent, and visible accountability throughout our organizations. Even though leaders can't make people respect each other, they can play a critical role in defining, promoting, and enforcing respectful behaviors.

A safe environment is the foundation for a positive workplace. Although the details will vary with each organization, leaders, and staff, there are four key principles that will support successful outcomes.

1. Build trust with ownership and long-term commitment.

2. Create explicit and consistent norms for interpersonal behavior.

3. Treat initial training *and* ongoing practice as equally important.

4. Enforce conduct at all levels.

Build Trust with Ownership and Long-term Commitment

Trust, once broken, is very difficult to rebuild. In many healthcare settings, trust has been broken again and again. This issue must be recognized if we are going to encourage the risk-taking required to make lasting changes in our workplace dynamics. Time, patience, and consistent new experiences will be necessary in order to build trust.

One of the most important, and often ignored, steps an organization can take is to demonstrate some ownership of the problem. I understand that leaders may be reluctant to take this step. There may be concerns of liability, time constraints, and a belief that "what's done is done", which leads some to adopt a strategy that looks only toward the future.

While I can sympathize with this line of thinking, I encourage leaders to be creative about taking ownership rather than avoiding it. I am not suggesting that a huge amount of time or resources be devoted to bringing up old situations and rehashing them. However, some situations may require attention. This is a judgment call, which may involve Human Resources and/or legal advice.

I am suggesting that leadership look for a way to acknowledge current problems. This is an opportunity to demonstrate accountability and build credibility around commitment to real change. I believe that there are many different and creative ways to do this that will allow residual troubles to be addressed efficiently. For example, a hospital CEO might send the message via meeting, letter, or video to all staff and doctors who practice in the facility. Such a letter could include:

- ✓ A commitment to a new way of being and an organizational plan of action.

- ✓ An acknowledgement that there may be parties who have intentionally or unintentionally ignored, witnessed, and/or participated in inappropriate behaviors in the past.

- ✓ An apology and request for forgiveness for any harm that has occurred and recognition that disrespectful treatment was never appropriate.

- ✓ A willingness to listen to old wounds with an appeal to go forward. (Employee assistance counselors and/or Human Resource personnel could strategize a way to hear and honor those who need support.)

This is a hard and very powerful step to take, but it will show staff that there is an honest and genuine resolve for new ways of being. It is an opportunity to role-model ownership and develop trust.

Create Explicit and Consistent Norms for Interpersonal Behavior

Norms are social rules that may be explicitly or implicitly stated. No organization explicitly allows abuse, but such behaviors have become ingrained in many of our workplaces. Consequently, we need explicit guidelines.

Norms provide a clear and visible definition of what is appropriate and expected professional behavior. Some organizations list respectful communications as part of a values statement, and others may have units develop their own list.

> *The best way to predict the future is to create it.*
>
> **--Peter Drucker**

Look for opportunities to invite input into the development of guidelines. An organization could develop an overarching mandate that requires respectful communication from all staff. Departments or units could then develop the specific guidelines that define this mandate. They may be called rules or "ways-of-being."

Such a list may look like this:

Ways-of-Being on Six West

- ✓ Provide direct feedback.

- ✓ Listen respectfully.

- ✓ Speak up assertively.

- ✓ Be open to other perspectives.

- ✓ Ensure kind and honest interactions.

- ✓ Allow room for learning.

- ✓ Use respectful non-verbal language.

This unit's norms could be posted in the nurses' lounge so they are visible at team meetings, and could also be put on a meeting agenda for revisions, recommitments, or for any time that members lead or join the team. We know from experience that the more participation there is from staff in developing the norms, the more invested they will be in them.

There are many options that a healthcare facility can consider when building norms. They can be part of orientation and can be included in the facility's handbook. I recommend that norms become a part of all administrative and medical staff contracts. If one physician or one CEO is allowed to be disrespectful, this will reflect a double standard and, in my opinion, will be the "kiss of death" to a change initiative of this nature.

Treat Initial Training and Ongoing Practice as Equally Important

Communication skill building and practice is as important as any clinical skill, especially when considering long-term quality, safety, and morale consequences. This training gives us an intellectual foothold on these practices and is an important beginning. Training in assertiveness and listening will provide baseline knowledge and should be provided for everyone.

Integrating these skills into everyday interactions will require practice and patience. Learning curves will vary with experience, motivation, stress, culture, and history. The trick here is to maintain clear, consistent, and enforced expectations while leaving room for making mistakes, forgiveness, and developing new relationships.

There will be times during emergency or high-stress procedures where tempers flare and new behaviors are more challenging to practice. In the middle of an emergency tracheotomy, it may not be realistic to give feedback about inappropriate behavior. However, making time to review behavior after the procedure and expecting different behavior the next time **is** important and realistic.

Receiving feedback in the form of "I" statements or other assertive language is often the first time offending individuals learn how their behaviors are impacting others. Giving and receiving feedback and relationship-building are tough and critical skills. They are a part of the skill development process that must continue after any formal training program. Support to ensure that this happens can be instilled all along an organization's hierarchy.

Some examples of support can include printed and posted materials on standard communication practices, creating or modifying a list of value statements that include respectful communication behaviors, integrating and/or refining communication skills into job evaluation protocols, and publicizing successes when both parties are willing. A senior administration, physician, or nursing leader who is willing to apologize for a disruptive behavior and share his/her learning in a newsletter or staff meeting could provide extremely powerful role-modeling and personal growth.

Recently, a workshop participant shared a story of how a physician was shocked when she told him that she felt intimidated by his behavior and realized that she was avoiding contact with him. She further stated that their relationship had drastically improved since she approached him.

Examples of standard communication such as the following guidelines for giving and receiving feedback could be included with the GRRRR model of listening in an organizational handbook for respectful communication. Notice how speaking up assertively is consistent with giving feedback and respectful listening is consistent with receiving it!

General Guidelines for Giving Feedback

- ✓ **Be kind and helpful.** Check in with your own intentions about offering feedback. Helping someone grow and learn is much different than issuing a put-down.

- ✓ **Check to see if feedback is desired.** Keep in mind that timing and location are crucial. *I have some feedback for you. Are you open to hearing it?* (If no, respect the person's decision). If you are in a leadership position and giving feedback that you must give, don't offer an option. If there is room for choice around time and place, it can be helpful to honor those.

√ **Be specific and don't judge or exaggerate.** Describe what you want to feed back without using words that indicate judgment. Don't use labels and don't exaggerate. Avoid loaded expressions such as "never" or "always."

√ **Ask questions.** In addition to sharing your thoughts, ask the person his/her opinion. Allow the receiver to suggest changes in behavior before offering options you may have.

√ **Perception check.** Ask questions to see if your message has been accurately heard, remembering that the message sent is not always the message received. You may need to present the feedback differently.

√ **Focus on your concern for the person and the behaviors which can be changed.** Monitor your attachment to "being right" or to the person changing in ways that you think s/he should.

General Guidelines for Receiving Feedback

√ **Breathe.** Remember you are a worthy person, separate from your actions and behaviors. Feedback is from the giver's perspective and you can choose what to receive.

√ **Listen carefully and try to drop your defensiveness.** Paraphrase the information you are receiving to make sure you understand the information. Validate the other person and ask questions for clarity.

√ **Acknowledge the feedback.** Let the person know you have heard him/her and that you will consider the feedback.

✓ **Take time to sort out what you have heard.** Give yourself time and space to assimilate and evaluate the information. Remember that it's not necessary to agree or disagree with the feedback. It is simply information. Let go of the need to justify, defend, or explain your actions. Don't over-internalize the feedback (i.e., assume it is all true).

✓ **Be honest with yourself.** Use feedback as an opportunity to create greater awareness. Explore any feelings created by the feedback.

✓ **Give yourself credit.** Receiving feedback can be hard work.

Enforce Conduct at All Levels

Although I am idealistic by nature and hope that everyone can and will learn respectful interactive skills, I realize that some may not. Ultimately, there must be a process of disciplinary action that holds staff, physician, nurse, and administrative leaders accountable. An organization that allows anyone to behave disrespectfully and continue to work or practice in the environment is giving that person permission to do so.

Nurses who tell other nurses that they should develop a thick skin or not worry about the way they were treated are giving permission for disrespectful behaviors to continue. Even nurses who talk about other nurses or physicians behind their backs are being disrespectful.

In public school systems there is an anti-bullying principle that states: *There are no innocent bystanders.* Healthcare leaders at all levels can make sure this principle is a standard expectation. In order for individuals to report and/or object to disruptive behaviors, they must trust that organizations will respond to complaints and that individuals will be held accountable.

Termination of job or loss of hospital privileges are last resorts, but must be real consequences for individuals who continue to display inappropriate behavior. It is a very difficult decision to hold a high-profile surgeon accountable for tirades in the OR or a 20-year nurse veteran for bullying on the unit. Yet these behaviors are impacting quality, safety, and morale beyond measure. Any genuine effort to stop them must include disciplinary procedures. Enforcing new behaviors with patients will require addressing additional issues, such as security and staffing, and will become much easier as we become adept at respectful interactions!

Summary

Once the message is clear and the consequences are credible, the toxic behaviors will stop, one way or another. Some folks will be open to reflecting on feedback and be grateful for it, even if it's painful. Some will be defensive, maybe even angry. There is always the possibility of negative responses, especially when new standards

> *Some men see things as they are and ask "Why?" I dream things that never were and ask, "Why not?"*
>
> **--Robert F. Kennedy**

are emerging. Things may get worse before they get better, and fears about retaliation are understandable. Enforcement of a new standard of behaviors is a critical element.

A safe and trusting environment is a crucial part of a foundation that supports and creates positive workplaces for everyone. Truly collaborative teams and organizations hold infinite promise for improving healthcare delivery and the practice of nursing. This can happen most efficiently and effectively when both individuals and organizations are working together towards this goal. The potential long-term benefit is profound.

We are close to the final, and perhaps most exciting, part of this book – where theory, insights, and skills become tools we can use to create positive workplaces.

Discussion Questions

1. What adjectives would you use to describe the ideal organizational culture in healthcare?

2. What challenges do you believe leaders face in creating this type of culture?

3. Why is trust such an important factor in developing a collaborative culture? What ideas do you have for rebuilding trust?

4. What do you suppose would happen to the communication in an organization that provides extensive training in assertiveness and listening, but does not enforce infractions?

Reflection Questions

1. How would you have felt if you were in my shoes when my supervisor asked me about the Lovenox injections? What about when the patient's wife told me that her husband always yelled at healthcare workers?

2. Have you ever experienced or witnessed an aggressive situation that involved a physician, supervisor or administrative leader? Do you remember how you felt? Can you describe the impact on your ability to think well?

3. Have you ever worked as a nurse in a positive workplace? How would you describe the culture at this workplace?

Part III: From Toxic to Positive Workplaces

Overview

In Part III, the theories, skills, and insights from Parts I and II come to fruition as we integrate them in the context of real nursing experiences. In the next two chapters, we will use case stories involving common toxic behaviors to discuss old and new ways of being. Each culminates with a revised account that paints a clear and hopeful picture of the positive workplaces we can create. The final chapter offers a realistic and encouraging message for moving forward together, despite the fact that we are all in different places!

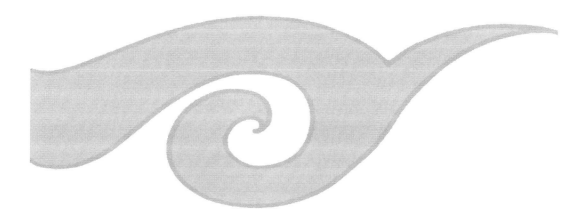

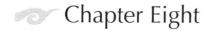 Chapter Eight

Connie's Story

Connie's Story

> *Being the new nurse on any job can be a difficult*
> *adjustment, but, in my experience, being the new nurse in*
> *the ED is brutal! I am 51 years old, with 30 years experience*
> *as an ED nurse. Most recently, I spent 11 years in a large city*
> *hospital emergency department.*

Thirty years of emergency room nursing! What a huge accomplishment!
I can only imagine the variety of clinical challenges this nurse has had.
What a wealth of knowledge she must have acquired, not to mention the
incredible heartache and stress she has experienced.

Connie's Story continued

> *As I look back over of my last four jobs, the orientation and*
> *assimilation process was torturous in each case. Most*
> *recently, my family and I had moved from New England to*
> *the Midwest, where I had accepted a job as an ED nurse in*
> *one of the two big city hospitals.*

Making the decision to create positive workplaces involves long-term
personal, professional, and organizational commitments. Stopping old
habits, taking risks, practicing new skills, making mistakes, and growing
and sharing power in new ways are all scary – and expected – parts of the
journey.

Connie's Story continued

> *During my two-month orientation period, I was ignored, misinformed, and generally treated like crap. My years of experience didn't matter. I was a new face in the ED and was subject to criticism and disdain as if it were my very first day as a nurse. I would say hello to staff members, and they wouldn't answer.*

I believe that we all need and deserve to have some power in our work. When we don't, or perceive that we don't, we look for indirect and often counterproductive ways to have a voice. Resistance to change, burnout, and/ or bullying are all-too-common examples in our profession.

> *The emotional brain responds to an event more quickly than the thinking brain.*
>
> **--Daniel Goleman**

Treating people with criticism and disdain sets a negative tone. New staff members and inexperienced nurses are less threatening, easy targets. The new nurse, even with years of valuable experience, won't know where to find things or who is responsible for what duties. For those of us with self-esteem issues, a passive or passive-aggressive welcome like this will surely chip away at our confidence and morale. When people are oppressed, it seems as though they can only find power in oppressing others. Even Connie seems to think that the treatment she was receiving would make more sense if it were her very first day as a nurse.

Of course, we don't know the details of this situation and, despite the fact that Connie feels mistreated, her colleagues may not intend to make her feel this way. Connie's perspective is legitimate, of course, but she would be wise to use caution in how she defines her colleagues' intentions. While it is entirely possible that they are mistreating her, it is also possible that they are exhausted, burned-out, and/or have very different personalities. Maybe a "hello" wasn't heard or perhaps Connie is soft-spoken. The truth is that we don't know what someone else's intentions are until they tell us or we ask. This is a potential opportunity for Connie to create an "I" statement to address the situation of colleagues who appear to be ignoring her. *Hey you guys, I'm feeling a little anxious as the new kid on the block. Did anyone hear me? I'd really like to be included.*

This is a non-threatening approach expressing ownership and an invitation for change. Maybe one or more colleagues will respond and make more of an effort. If not, then, at the very least, Connie will have a clear idea, early on, about the challenges she will be facing. Further, this idea will be grounded in the reality of her current situation and not informed by previous experiences or assumptions. Finding ways to cope and work with these individuals will be key. Also, this approach will provide a great gauge for determining with whom she may want to build friendships.

Making a new staff member feel welcome should be an organizational priority, and it sounds as if there is room for improvement on this unit. We will consider this again as the story unfolds.

Connie's Story continued

Leah, another ED RN, seemed to have it in for me. One day, I was reluctant to go to lunch because I feared a patient was internally bleeding, and the ED doctor did not seem concerned. I had suggested some lab work, which he ordered. I was anxious for the results and wanted to make sure any abnormal values were immediately brought to his attention. Leah encouraged me to go to lunch and promised to keep an eye out for the results.

While in the cafeteria, I heard a code called in the ED. When I got back to the unit, my patient was being whisked off to the OR. The ED doc reamed me out for not reporting the critical lab values immediately. I looked at Leah and she said, "The lab just called a minute ago." I would have believed her, but when I saw her exchange a half smile and shoulder shrug with the Unit Coordinator it made me wonder. When I expressed my frustration to another staff RN, her reply was, "I guess everybody has to earn their stripes."

It is mind boggling how many common communication and relationship issues are potentially going on in this scenario. In each issue, there are opportunities to use the skills presented in this book.

Connie thinks the physician isn't concerned about the patient's possible internal bleeding. How does she, or would she, know this? Is there room for this physician to teach and/or learn something here? She is worried enough to assert the need for blood work, and he is receptive to ordering it. This suggests that some collaborative teamwork is going on.

> *I don't think you ever stop giving. I really don't. I think it's an on-going process. And it's not just about being able to write a check. It's being able to touch somebody's life.*
>
> **--Oprah Winfrey**

I wonder if Connie realizes that her 30 years of nursing have provided her with an experience base that makes her concern an extremely valuable asset. Maybe even the physician realizes this. In fact, what if he ordered the lab work because of it? Has either of these professionals ever said anything to each other about mutual respect? How would a quick *Thanks for suggesting it* from the physician and/or *Thanks for considering my input* from Connie help to build on this collaboration? As they begin to share a little more of their experience, the foundation for a respectful relationship can grow. So often miscommunication arises when we assume what other people are thinking or feeling and use our assumptions to guide our responses.

What if Connie had been direct with him? Could her assumption about his concern be turned into a teaching opportunity? What if she were to say something like, *Hey Dr. Jones, I'm really worried that this guy is bleeding internally and going to crash. My sense is that you are not concerned. Can you share your thinking with me?* This approach creates an opportunity for the physician to learn how his demeanor appears to Connie, allows him to reconsider his patient's status, and helps set the scene for a more collaborative working relationship.

It also paves the way for, *I'm headed to lunch and have reported off to Leah.* Thus the accountability issue is addressed in terms of quality and safety rather than getting lost in toxic relationships. Leah, with the appropriate training and support, will also have the option of saying, *I can't cover for you, Connie, I've got blood running and there is an MVA en route.* If nobody can cover for Connie, it may not be a good time for her to go to lunch. If this happens frequently, then staffing issues can come into focus. By setting limits and respecting them, other problems become clearer.

Missing meals is another complex and common problem among nurses. A nurse manager from a med/surg unit recently asked me how I would apply my recommendations to a situation where the Human Resources department had issued a new policy mandating meal breaks. She believed her staff was getting around the policy by using their time cards to punch out and back in for a meal break, but continuing to work.

We discussed how unhealthy this strategy was for nurses, patients, and the facility. I encouraged her to look for ways to invite input from individual nurses and representatives from Human Resources. For instance, the staff nurses could ask themselves or (be asked) such questions as:

1. What is preventing me from taking breaks?

2. What do I need in order to take breaks?

3. What questions could I ask Human Resources in order to understand their perspective?

Meanwhile, human resource staff could consider some similar questions such as:

1. What is the impact on HR when nurses don't take meal breaks?

2. What do nurses need from HR to increase compliance?

3. What limits does HR have regarding the new policy?

The current strategy of punching out and continuing to work seems like a power struggle without much understanding of each other's perspectives. Asking questions such as these could help both sides come to mutual understanding and, from there, develop some creative ideas.

Some organizations may truly want to support the need for nurses to take meal breaks, while others may be content to look the other way. Also, some nurses may get some secondary gains from repeatedly missing breaks. Saving the day, feeling victimized, avoiding the risk of setting limits are all possibilities. If both sides are willing to be accountable for their part and respectful of each other's needs, it is much more likely that realistic solutions will emerge. Who knows, perhaps they'll develop a new part-time break-nurse position or differential, obtain training on assertiveness, or pilot some new scheduling model.

Also, let's keep in mind the realities of working in a busy emergency department. Is it possible that Connie's patient is in a critical situation despite all the good work from the physician, nurses, lab staff, and others? How is this likely to affect the team?

Of course, it is possible that Leah knew about the lab results and purposefully delayed reporting them. This, as we all know, is alarming and certainly grounds for negligence – something both she and the organization should take very seriously.

The doctor, according to Connie, "reamed her out." He may have anger management issues or a hearing problem that leads to a loud voice. He may be knowingly abusive in a hospital that has tolerated his behavior for years, and he may not realize how his behavior is impacting others. Until someone is willing to offer him feedback, he may remain clueless about how his demeanor affects others. In my opinion, we owe each other the opportunity to grow and learn from feedback. The situation is more complicated with differences in power, and being safe is always the priority. All the more reason to create safe environments!

Next, a colleague dismisses Connie's experience with her remark about "earning stripes." What if, instead, she had said something like, *Wow, that sounds frustrating. I'm sorry that you had that experience. How can I help?* This validation doesn't solve the problem, but it does honor

Connie's feelings and leaves room for her to invite support.

In our work in healthcare, there are times when, no matter how much we do and how effectively we do it, people will still code and/or die. This causes extraordinary stress, and we are all trying to deal with it. Finding ways and resources for expressing grief and frustration without these painful blaming games is crucial. Really, we are in this together.

> *The last of the human freedoms is to choose one's attitude in any given set of circumstances.*
>
> **--Victor Frankl**

Connie's Story continued

> *Another time, Leah was talking and laughing with a colleague. As I walked up to them, they suddenly became silent. When I asked them what they were laughing about, Leah rolled her eyes and muttered something to the other nurse as they turned their backs to me and walked away.*

This is a classic example of covert horizontal violence. It is extremely challenging to address and is extremely destructive to workplace relationships. It is imperative to stop it.

There are a couple of options that Connie might consider in terms of directly dealing with this situation. Depending on her comfort level, she might speak up at the moment. *Wait a minute you guys. I'm confused about what just happened. It seemed to me that your talking and laughing stopped abruptly when I joined you. When I asked you about it, you rolled your eyes, and Leah said something to Sue that I couldn't hear. I feel excluded and wonder if you were talking about me or laughing at me for some reason. What's going on?*

Another option would be to ask each of these nurses later for a few minutes to clarify something or offer feedback, perhaps in a quieter space after work, where they can talk without distractions. This allows for more separate, and possibly safer, one-to-one conversations. The sooner Connie resolves this, the better. Even if Leah was being disrespectful and won't, or can't, admit it, both she and her colleague will soon learn that Connie will speak up about her concerns. This adds a predictable consequence to their behavior that they may keep in mind for future interactions. Remember, Connie cannot make Leah respect her, but she can insist on being treated respectfully.

This scenario also brings up the issue of friendships at work and working relationships. There can be room for both, but some guidelines are important. Working relationships require that we get the job done and help each other according to patient needs and clinical standards. We must behave respectfully towards one other with these objectives in mind whether we like each other or not.

Developing friendships at work is a natural occurrence and a wonderful benefit of working together, whereas triangles and alliances can create negative working relationships. We must be mindful of how friendships may impact the team and nurture them at appropriate times and places.

In this situation, it is possible that Leah and her colleague have a longstanding friendship and were discussing something that had nothing to do with Connie. They are certainly entitled to their private relationship, but they would do well to have that conversation in private later, or might at least offer a quick apology and look for a way to include Connie in their conversation. *Sorry, Connie, we were having a private conversation. I can understand how it might appear to you, but we weren't talking about or laughing at you. How was your weekend off?* Again, this dance of ownership and listening can lead to new understandings and behaviors.

Connie's Story continued

> *I decided to talk with my manager, Valerie, about this and similar incidents. I ended up crying in her office. She told me she knew that Leah could be "hard on new people" and that "her bark was worse than her bite." She assured me that "deep down inside, Leah had a heart of gold and was a crackerjack nurse." She encouraged me to "give it some more time" and told me that I was "showing some great potential, but should try not to be so sensitive." I felt awful leaving her office.*

Connie reaches out for some support from her supervisor who basically tells her that she is aware of Leah's behaviors and is excusing them. This gives Leah permission to continue bullying and sends a message to Connie and other staff that the organization will support Leah in her behaviors and not support attempts to stop it. Her suggestion that Connie be less sensitive is another way of condoning inappropriate behavior and ultimately twists it around so that Connie is to blame because she is too sensitive.

What a mess! Leah may have been negligent and seems to have a history of non-verbal abuse, the physician is angry at Connie, Connie is frustrated with everyone, and the nursing supervisor keeps the toxic dynamics going.

Connie's Story continued

> Over the next few weeks, I dreaded going to work and started to feel very depressed and lonely. I had no mentor, and no one even offered to help me adjust. A nurse who had started two weeks after I did ended up quitting within one month. I can only wonder why? I am not happy in my job, but my family needs the income. I am not sure where I'll be a year or two from now. Maybe here, maybe not.

It is pretty tough to expect one nurse to change the dynamics in this department. Some of you reading this book might be thinking that you'd be alone in this work, and the prospects for real change are questionable. I understand. You are the best judge of what risks you can take.

The following scenario demonstrates what might happen when one nurse moves forward despite a work culture that doesn't.

A New Version for Connie

> I was confused after meeting with Valerie. I felt as if she was supporting me in some ways and not in others. She accepted Leah's behavior, and I felt I had to as well. I knew I wouldn't go back to her with any similar problem. I survived the first six months. I dreaded going to work and seldom

went to lunch. I became more and more aware of how unhappy I was.

I got some support from a mental health counselor. This helped me cope with my work life, understand myself, and ultimately look for a way out. I decided to take advantage of the hospital's tuition reimbursement program and was accepted into a graduate program in Healthcare Administration. I cut back my hours as much as I could and made friends with some nurses who had also "survived."

In school, I found that I was especially interested in courses about organizational communication, conflict, and leadership. I began to study and understand some of the interpersonal dynamics that were prevalent in my current and previous nursing positions.

I had many opportunities to practice assertiveness and feedback techniques in the ED at my hospital. Unfortunately, I didn't feel as if I was able to make much of a dent in the kinds of passive and passive-aggressive behaviors that I was becoming adept at recognizing.

I became more and more frustrated with the lack of professionalism and even found myself being rude at times. I remember feeling ashamed of giving the cold shoulder to a traveling RN who was filling a much-needed position. Although I apologized after reflecting on my behavior, I realized I was feeling hopeless about the unit and my ability to practice new skills in a healthy way.

As I neared the end of my graduate program, I responded to an ad for a nurse management position in the ED of the other city hospital.

During my interview, I discovered that this organization was in the second year of promoting a very progressive program on anti-bullying. The Director of HR said the CEO had insisted upon a hospital-wide policy of zero tolerance of abuse. He informed me that when the policy was announced it was followed with training for all staff, including senior management. When I asked for specifics about the training, I learned that it included identifying covert and overt abuse and assertiveness and that, if hired, I would be required to take the same training as part of my orientation process. He told me that the culture was changing, but was not perfect yet.

When I was called back for a second interview, I was asked how I would handle a situation where a new nurse reported covert bullying by a veteran nurse.

I took a deep breath and exhaled slowly, "First, I would like to know more about where the unit was in terms of the culture shift and what hospital protocols were in place. I would want to validate the new nurse's experience, probe for details of the incident, and thank her for coming forward. If it felt safe, I might suggest direct feedback using "I" statements. If the nurse did not feel safe, or the unit was in the early phases of change, I would want to be more directly involved in the process. I believed that, as a manager, I would need to be a visible and reliable proponent of the new policy. I would want to find out more about the other nurse's perspective as well as that of any bystanders. This might lead to a facilitated meeting of the key players. I would seek support from HR and upper level nursing management. Options that I would consider would be job-coaching, more training for individuals and the team, and, if necessary, disciplinary action."

I knew this would be hard work for everyone involved, but the idea of working through this conflict with a leadership vision that I felt aligned with was very exciting.

I was thrilled to accept their offer!

Summary

Optimizing workplace culture and practicing assertiveness and respectful listening will go a long way towards improving workplace dynamics, yet this is much more of an art than a science. In the real world, communication is messy. Our feelings may be hurt, assumptions and presumptions may go untested, and we may have fears of repercussions and/or develop skills in faultfinding.

Companies used to be able to function with autocratic bosses. We don't live in that world anymore.

--Rosabeth Moss Kanter

My students and workshop participants present great examples of challenging situations, often hoping I will offer simple and clear problem-solving instructions. Only rarely do I have such magic bullets. More often I lead discussions which shed light on how the skills and insights we are talking about will contribute to solutions. I'm happy to give examples of how I might handle a problem, but I never tell them how they should respond, since their personal concerns, history, and other perspectives are part of the mix, as are variations in skill level and support.

I do encourage them to look for opportunities where these skills could be developed, applied, and supported. I also help them reflect on how they may be contributing to a tough situation. Honestly, in the course of gaining expertise in this work, I have learned much about my own contributions to difficult dynamics over the years.

The more we understand ourselves and seek to understand each other, the more we contribute to healthy workplace dynamics. Realistically, one nurse in a toxic environment may face the need to cope with it or leave. Neither situation is optimal, and both are very personal, and possibly difficult, decisions.

I find it hopeful that there is a growing concern about the nursing shortage, that initiatives are in place to eliminate abuse, and that there is a developing awareness of the need for practicing effective communication.

In the next chapter, we'll look at an aggressive physician in a passive culture and how things can evolve when individuals and organizations are held responsible for respectful communication from every angle.

Discussion Questions

1. Brainstorm a list of reasons why nurses might skip meal breaks.

2. What ideas do you have that would help nurses to take scheduled breaks more regularly?

3. What thoughts do you think nurses have when a new nurse with lots of experience from another job joins their unit?

4. How do you think Connie felt when her colleague told her that "everyone has to earn their stripes"?

5. What ideas do you have for Connie if she had not been offered a new position?

Reflection Questions:

1. Describe some of the different friendships that you have at work? After reading this chapter, do you see any need to be more careful about excluding others or finding private space for private relationships?

2. Briefly describe a situation that you experienced or observed that involved covert and/ or horizontal violence. What might you have done differently, given the skills and insights from this book or other resources? What could someone in a leadership position have done differently?

Chapter Nine

Nancy's Story

Nancy's Story

> *I was working day shift, and my patient had been taken down for a colonoscopy just before my shift started. As I got out of report, I was confronted by the gastroenterologist, Dr. Smith, who had left the patient sedated in the GI suite to come to my floor and yell at me for sending her down when she wasn't "cleaned out." It was in the middle of the hallway, with several co-workers and other doctors around. He was screaming in my face about how stupid I was for sending her down, not giving me a chance to tell him I didn't send her. I was stunned at first, then embarrassed, and then angry. I had only been a nurse for a short period of time and did end up crying after he left. This was this particular doctor's M.O., so, I didn't feel there was anything I could do. I did write him up anyway. It made me feel a little better, but I didn't hear anything from it.*

I can't help but wonder how this interaction, lasting probably less than a minute, affected her relationship with this doctor, her feelings about herself, the unit, the nursing profession, and the organization for a long time to come. It is as if the playground bully grew up and became a doctor, and other staff, including physicians, continued to tacitly tolerate his behavior.

I remember a similar incident early in my own career. I was in my first two weeks of practice on a med/surg unit. I was assessing a patient's IV that had infiltrated when a surgeon stormed in the room and asked me what the hell I was doing. I remember feeling shocked and flustered. What had I done wrong? I probably was too anxious to sort out all that I was feeling, but I imagine that, somewhere in the mix, I was blaming myself for his bad behavior. Maybe I was an awful nurse or an incompetent one. Maybe I was angry about the way he treated me in front of this patient. I'm sure I was humiliated. That was over 20 years ago. I told no one.

> *When people act against other people, they feel justified. They feel sensible. If an act against a person is justified in the mind of the perpetrator, it is, in a backwards way, said to be caused by the victim rather than by the perpetrator. Just the opposite of the truth.*
>
> **--Patricia Evans**

Recently, in a workshop I was giving on understanding and improving workplace dynamics, there were three staff nurses from the same hospital. They shared how one physician in particular was notorious for yelling at nurses and how they all cringed when they heard his voice on the unit. One nurse shared that she dreaded calling him about patient issues because he had a tendency to mumble questions and orders, and when she tried to clarify what he was saying, he would get mad and yell.

Think about this. The doctor mumbles about what he wants and then gets mad at the nurse (or seems to), when the nurse isn't clear about what he wants. This is a set up for failure, and the nurse an easy target for abuse.

Compounded by self-esteem issues that the nurse may have and an organizational culture that tolerates it, such toxic behaviors continue unabated.

Anger, fear, anxiety, and a sense of dread are all common feelings regarding interactions with a person who has exhibited abusive behaviors.

Consider how much power this physician has and how unhealthy this dynamic is. In terms of numbers, the percentage of professionals in this community who treat nurses or others this way is probably small, but this one person's behaviors have enormous and wide spread repercussions. Dr. Smith's M.O. is well known, and many are afraid of him.

In my classes and workshops on leadership, organizational communication, and conflict, discussions often include nurses from one or two facilities who will share stories that lead to others from the same organization acknowledging similar experiences with the same individual. It seems as if there is always at least one person who is notorious for bad behavior.

In Nancy's story, she took the step to report Dr. Smith and never heard anything back. This essentially gives him permission to behave this way and robs him of the chance to grow as a human being.

> *Aggression unopposed becomes a contagious disease.*
>
> **--Jimmy Carter**

Abuse has never been explicitly condoned, but it has been implicitly accepted. What I mean is that no organization has ever stated its approval for doctors to be aggressive or nurses to be passive-aggressive. No hospital that I know of has a policy that states, "We have a partial tolerance for abuse!" That would be absurd, and yet it is basically true. This long history of mixed messages is partly why this is such a tough problem to solve.

I first read about the term, "zero tolerance for abuse" in The Joint Commission *Guide to Improving Staff Communication* that was published in 2005. Four years later, in January 2009, The Joint Commission's new requirement for addressing disruptive behavior goes into effect.[22] This new standard includes requirements for establishing a code of conduct and a process for managing inappropriate behaviors. In addition, The Joint Commission goes on to provide a comprehensive list of suggested actions regarding educating, enforcing, and documenting related issues.

Even with recent press and efforts by such organizations as The Joint Commission, Institute of Healthcare Improvement, and the National Association for Healthcare Quality, there is reluctance to fully acknowledge the depth and breadth of this problem. In her article, "Hospital Bullies Take a Toll on Patient Safety," health writer JoNel Aleccia quotes the president of the American Medical Association, Dr. Joseph Heyman , "I don't see it as a huge problem," he said. "Having standards encourages hospitals to look for this kind of behavior and head it off at the pass."

This kind of attitude perpetuates the confusion that surrounds toxic behaviors. How do we get nurses to actively set limits or report abuse if some of the primary perpetrators are the ones with the

---

22 *For more information, visit The Joint Commission website home page under Sentinel Events and then Sentinel Event Alerts. Look for issue 40 – July 9, 2008: "Behaviors that undermine a culture of safety."*

most positional power and their colleagues "don't see it as a huge problem"?

Organizations have a rich opportunity here. As they develop policies and procedures to meet TJC's requirement or develop their own initiatives, they can look for ways to show ownership for old unhealthy dynamics and their commitment to new healthy ones. One way to do this would be to offer an announcement from senior management that includes an acknowledgement and apology about the past and a request to move forward. This does not need to be a long and involved probe into old wounds. Such a letter might look like this:

Dear ABC Hospital Staff,

As your CEO, I am writing to prepare ABC Hospital for its policy of ZERO tolerance for abuse. This policy goes into effect immediately and includes a long-term plan for related training and enforcement. This letter is the first of many important steps.

We are learning how pervasive disruptive behaviors are in healthcare workplaces, and our facility is no exception. I realize that there may be individuals who have experienced disrespectful treatment in the past, and I want to publicly apologize for any inappropriate behaviors that have occurred in this workplace.

No one deserves to be treated disrespectfully. I am sorry for any such behavior experienced by staff at this facility. I cannot erase the past, but I can acknowledge it and offer resources to help build a better future.

If you have been a target of, or have witnessed, disruptive behaviors here or in other healthcare facilities and would like to share your experience openly, please contact Human Resources. If you would prefer anonymous support, please contact the Employee Assistance Program we have set up to help with this initiative.

I urge you to join me in creating a culture where we can work safely and respectfully together and offer the highest in healthcare quality.

Sincerely,

A powerful memo like this could go a long way toward building trust and, with it, help set the stage for identifying, reporting, and stopping toxic behaviors. Even the most skeptical of nurses might begin to believe that things can and will be different. Seeking input for creatively taking this step from nursing staff, Human Resources, medical and administrative leadership, and others will likely increase investment in change as well as demonstrate accountability, credibility, and sincerity.

Perhaps this is not a measure that all organizations will or should take. There may be liability issues or other concerns which leadership must consider before acting on this suggestion. In any case, getting the idea on the table seems like a valuable opportunity for discussion!

This shift in dynamics will be stressful on many. It will not happen overnight and there will be resistance. Nevertheless, moving forward is crucial. How would such a situation play out if there was a fully functional "zero tolerance for abuse"? In the following rewrite of Nancy's story, you will see how all members of the team play a role in sustaining a culture that clearly promotes and enforces respectful communication.

A New Version of Nancy's Story

He was screaming in my face about how stupid I was for sending her down, not giving me a chance to say anything. I put my hands out with arms slightly bent and palms about half way up while pivoting slightly to the side[23] and said, "Stop yelling at me. I do not deserve this treatment."

> *I will not allow myself to be less than I am to meet anyone's expectations.*
>
> **--Unknown**

Another physician standing by approached Dr. Smith, "You're out of line, Joe. Take 5 minutes and cool off." Dr. Smith paused and stepped back as Nancy continued, "I will help address your concerns when you talk to me respectfully."

The Nurse Manager overheard the incident and immediately came over, "Are you OK, Nancy? We will follow-up regarding this inappropriate conversation later. In the

---

23 *This is known as the "mediator's stance." In addition to using a clear and firm voice, body language for such a face-to-face confrontation defines your personal space without blocking the aggressive person. In a sense you get out of their way and still maintain a non-defensive, non-threatening, and strong posture.*

meantime, who is the patient? I will call GI and either reschedule or address procedure preparation needs now."

Dr. Smith returned to the GI suite. Others resumed working. Nancy took a few minutes to collect herself and then did the same.

The nursing supervisor solved the immediate crisis with respect to the patient and put the topic of GI preparation on the agenda for the next team meeting in addition to addressing the concern with the nursing supervisor on the night shift. The potential for team problem-solving would be included in discussions.

Later in the shift, the nursing supervisor helped Nancy fill out an incident report and made sure she was feeling supported. Human Resources arranged to facilitate a follow-up discussion involving Nancy, the nursing supervisor, and Dr. Smith within 72 hours.

In this meeting Nancy was able to express how Dr. Smith's behavior impacted her. She felt supported by her supervisor and HR. She used "I" statements to explain that when he was yelling at her and stepping into her personal space she felt afraid, anxious, and humiliated. She warned him that she would not stay present if he behaved in such a way again, and that she expected him to follow the hospital's communication protocols.

Dr. Smith validated her feelings and assured her that he would not treat her disrespectfully again. He shared that he had been called into surgery at 3 a.m. the morning of the incident, and his patient had died on the operating room table. Nancy indicated that she could understand his stress and exhaustion and could imagine how frustrated he must have been.

All in the meeting acknowledged that the issue about patient prep did not in any way justify the physician's abuse. The nursing supervisor committed to working with her team to minimize future occurrences. Dr. Smith offered to be a resource. Nancy accepted his apology. She knew that time and new experiences with him would help to restore trust. She would remain cautious, but with support from leadership in all areas, she was open to developing an effective and professional relationship with him.

This was the third reported incident for Dr. Smith in the last month. The hospital was holding him accountable, and he was beginning to realize that his explosive anger was impacting patients, nurses, and his career. In addition to his apology to Nancy, Dr. Smith privately discussed the situation with the medical director and made a commitment to seek anger management support.

The medical director provided him with appropriate referrals and asked him to check back in a week or two to discuss progress. The director shared that he had done some similar work a few years ago and had grown a great deal. He

167

offered that it was not easy, but that he believed it helped him grow as a person and physician. He offered that he would support him in any way he could. Dr. Smith was surprised to hear the medical director's experience dealing with anger management.

The medical director warned him that another incident of abusive behavior would result in disciplinary action. Dr. Smith made an appointment with an organizational psychologist who had special training in working with physicians in this area. He was angry, frustrated, ashamed, and relieved.

At this hospital, all clinical and administrative staff, including physicians, received training in assertiveness and respectful listening. In addition, the CEO has implemented a hospital-wide standard for respectful communication. There really is a zero tolerance for abuse in this facility and everyone knows it. Resources are available through Human Resources to help staff develop and practice their skills including an Employee Assistance Program.

Summary

Nancy's stories provide a forum for comparing a system where all parties are contributing to a positive workplace with one where an aggressive hierarchy dominates. Evolving out of these old patterns requires a long-term commitment to changes that are difficult. Having a clear and hopeful vision of what things could be like can be a source of inspiration for taking steps, including some difficult ones, towards positive workplaces.

Discussion Questions

1. What reasoning do you think Dr. Joseph Heyman might have for thinking that bullying is not a big problem?

2. What would you like physicians to know about nurses' experiences with bullying in the workplace?

3. Does Jimmy Carter's quote about aggression make sense to you? Why or why not?

4. Consider your own workplaces and the new version of Connie's story. Which aspects ring true for your organization? Which areas could be opportunities for your workplace to do a better job?

Reflection Questions

1. What thoughts and feelings did you have when reading the sample CEO letter in this chapter? What difference would a note like this make to you if your organization was establishing a zero tolerance for abuse?

2. Briefly describe a situation that you experienced or observed that involved overt and/ or vertical violence. What might you have done differently given the skills and insights from this book or other resources? What could someone in a leadership position have done differently?

Chapter Ten

Champions for Change

Margaret J. Wheatley[24] describes a leader as "anyone who wants to help." I find her work compelling. She believes very strongly in the creative and problem-solving power of human relationships and collaboration. I believe that her definition of leadership includes all of us and that the more respectful our communication skills are, the healthier our relationships and the more productive our collaborations will be.

The cause-and-effect links from self-awareness, ownership, and respect for other perspectives to solutions about staffing, workplace violence, and safety, etc. are not always clear or direct. They are difficult to see at times, often hard to change, and maybe impossible to quantify. Consequently, they may be tempting to ignore. I urge you to look for them. They are there!

In healthcare we are trained to measure, predict, and contain. Many times this is exactly what we need to do to optimize outcomes, but not always! Creativity is illusive. We may know what it feels like and know that we want it,

> *Not everything that counts can be counted; and not everything that can be counted, counts.*
>
> **--Albert Einstein**

but we have trouble making it happen. This is, I believe, because

---

24 *To learn more about Margaret J. Wheatley, go to her website, (www.margaretwheatley.com). You will find articles, podcasts, and information about her books.*

creativity is something that is innate in us all and emerges from ourselves and in the light of our relationships. This can happen spontaneously and without inhibition when we feel safe.

One of the most exciting experiences I have as a teacher/trainer is facilitating opportunities for learning that lead to self awareness that in turn leads to more respectful communication practices. Just recently in a course I teach on leadership, one of my students was sharing her experience with an assignment involving an interview with a leader she admired. To complete this task, the students had to develop questions, meet with their interviewee, and write a report describing the conversation.

I had noticed some limitations with respect to this student's listening skills over the first few classes. I found that, as a facilitator, I was often intervening to address her tendencies to interrupt and make sweeping assumptions, and I nudged her to validate other perspectives. I could see that she was having a hard time accepting that other viewpoints were just as valid as hers and that, when different, were not putting hers in peril. I wasn't sure if we were making progress and listened intently as she described how exasperating she found the interview assignment.

> *I was trying my best to listen to what he was saying and take notes at the same time. It was really hard for me, and I was worried that I wasn't going to get everything. A couple of times I tried to summarize what he had said, so I asked him questions to see if I understood him. No, I didn't! I was shocked. I never realized how easy it was to misunderstand someone!*

174

She was incredulous at this gap between what she thought he meant and what he did mean! A light bulb was going on, and it was fun to see! Not only did she experience a new awareness about herself, but she also got to experience more effective communication! Eureka! She can learn from him more easily and completely now! It seems likely that there will be similar opportunities for her as she goes forward on her leadership path. Who knows how this might help bridge her knowledge, experience, and skill with new ideas?

Another current story involves Karen, a nurse manager with whom I work as a coach. She is considering approaching a physician in an effort to build their relationship. She describes to me a long history of working with Dr. Johnson. Their relationship, at least from her perspective, has evolved into a dynamic of chronic frustration, fear, and avoidance.

She uses an example of his writing illegibly, not being able to understand his orders, and being afraid to clarify, yet calling him because she knows she should, only to have him yell at her over the phone and insist that she should have known what he meant. Karen dreads working with him, wants a better relationship, and sees that there may be an opportunity to influence change.

Some of the work she is doing in our coaching sessions is focused on building her assertiveness. In our last phone conversation she described to me how she was thinking of addressing the situation. I asked her to verbalize how she might ask to meet with him, and how she might initiate a conversation about her concerns.

Her initial approach:

Dr. Johnson, I need to talk with you about our communication. When do you have time to sit down with me privately for 5 or 10 minutes in the next few days?

> *Freedom fighters don't always win, but they are always right.*
>
> **--Molly Ivins**

Her plan, if he agreed to meet with her:

Thanks for taking the time to meet with me and hear my concerns. I've been reading about assertiveness and am developing that skill. In the process, I've realized that some of our interactions over the years have had an unhealthy tone. I'm talking about phone and face-to-face conversations when I have called to clarify your orders and you seem to become angry and yell at me that I should know what you meant. I find now that I dread having to communicate with you. I know that this is not professional, and I'd like our communications to be respectful. What thoughts do you have?

She is unsure if she will take the steps she is describing. She is anxious that he will refuse to meet or if he meets, will deny her concerns, or worse yell at her for wasting his time. I understand and honor her caution. She has had experiences in her life with folks who are responsive to respectful communication and some who are not.

The hospital where she works is preparing new strategies regarding zero tolerance, and she is not sure if she should wait. Her language and ownership are clear, kind, open, and assertive. If she decides to take the risk with this physician and he is willing, there is great potential for him to learn how he is perceived on the unit and perhaps in other areas.

We are undergoing a sea change in healthcare, and shifting out of these chronic relationships will be difficult. Conversations like these are scary, especially with traditional power dynamics in place. Yet the rippling effect of such a dialogue has vast potential:

- ✓ The physician can experience growth in self-awareness in regards to his writing and phone demeanor.

- ✓ He has an opportunity to become a better leader and develop his own self-respect.

- ✓ The nurse and doctor can forge a new relationship where teaching and learning are ongoing components.

- ✓ Morale and job satisfaction can improve for this nurse and her colleagues.

- ✓ Everyone, including patients, will experience less stressful dynamics.

- ✓ There can be a decrease in errors due to miscommunication; quality and cost effectiveness improves.

There is no doubt in my mind that there will be some risk inherent in making the changes to positive workplaces. However, deciding when, where, and how to take these risks are very personal decisions – ones that we must respect, for each other and for ourselves. In this case, the doctor has a history of aggressive and passive-aggressive behavior with this nurse manager. She has a history of being somewhat passive and passive-aggressive with him, (i.e. by not calling him on his behavior and talking about him behind his back with her colleagues). She has new assertiveness skills to bring to the table, but no control over his willingness or capacity to listen.

> *No pessimist ever discovered the secret of the stars or sailed an uncharted land, or opened a new doorway for the human spirit.*
>
> **--Helen Keller**

Time will tell whether she goes forward with her strategy. I am excited about her ability to frame a potential meeting in such an assertive way. If he doesn't agree to meet with her, I will ask her to consider taking her concerns to her supervisor or Human Resources. I know that she will make the best decisions for her, based on the circumstances and her comfort level. I also trust that if she chooses to initiate a conversation with him, she will show ownership, confidence, and a willingness to collaborate.

Summary

In closing, I believe that you, too, will make the best decisions on how and when to use this material. The tools in this book will help you to make your best effort and at the same time set a higher standard for colleagues. Sometimes, and, I hope, often, this will result in inspiring others to meet you in a higher place. This is the place where creative and collaborative problem-solving promote happier, healthier workplaces.

Other times, putting your best foot forward may lead only to a clearer picture of the underlying issues stemming from particular people and/or cultures. You may not be able to influence these directly, or to the extent that you would like, but you will have a better understanding of what you are dealing with. Instead of possibly contributing to the dysfunction, you can focus on strategizing ways to optimize, cope with, or seek alternative experiences. This, too, is powerful progress.

We are all at different places in our lives with different circumstances to consider. Thinking about change, talking about new ways of being, and acting on thoughts and discussions are all vital contributions!

As a nurse, I already know that you are smart and compassionate. I trust that you will integrate the tools here when you are ready, when you find them appropriate, and when you sense the support of your organization. Each time you do, keep in mind that you are acting as a champion for change and that you will ultimately impact delivery of healthcare in your workplace and, quite possibly, on a more global scale.

Our workplaces can and should be positive, supporting environments where we practice our profession in an atmosphere of respect. As more and more of us set limits and insist on appropriate behavior, we will automatically become proactive partners in establishing reasonable workloads, cost-effective quality, safer care, and healthy work-life balances. Our confident voices can, and will, change the landscape of healthcare for the better.

Discussion Questions

1. Consider Einstein's quote in this chapter and discuss how this might be applied to healthcare.

2. If Karen decides not to ask Dr. Johnson to have a private conversation, what suggestions do you have that would help her to optimize or cope with the current situation?

3. Describe both positive and negative scenarios that could evolve if Karen talks with Dr. Johnson.

Reflection Questions

1. How would you feel about asking a physician or other leader to talk about a chronic problem relationship?

2. Who do you know who has worked in a positive healthcare environment? Write a list of questions you could ask this person that would show curiosity about communication, conflict management, and teams in that workplace.

3. Describe a work relationship that you would like to improve. What steps can you take to initiate a new dynamic?

4. Do you know someone who could be a resource for you as you use the tools and information in this book to develop your confident voice?

Epilogue: Where Nurses Nurture Their Young

I have been a nurse for thirty years and remember in the 1980's when the catchphrase "nurses eat their young" came out. I couldn't understand why good nurses would choose to not support the younger, less experienced nurses and help them become the best healthcare providers they could be. This pervasive attitude has continued to move throughout healthcare and needs to be examined and corrected.

Later, after I received my MNSc in Nursing Administration and started teaching, it amazed me to hear of nurses who told nursing students that they were "wasting their time" that nursing was a "thankless profession." I became curious as to why this change has grown and nurses are less satisfied with their professions. After reviewing a working draft of *Confident Voices*, I found that Beth offers us refreshing insight into this troublesome issue. In addition to helping us understand workplace dynamics, nurses are encouraged to discuss issues that are happening in the workplace and are given the tools to do so with ownership and respect.

Verbalizing a stressful or fearful situation to supportive people is a great way to debrief a volatile situation and help resolution come about more therapeutically to the nurse and staff. It is essential that nurses feel they have a safe environment in which to discuss fears and feelings without judgment and reprisals in order to remain content and productive in their profession.

I am currently in a doctoral program and have chosen violence/aggression in nursing as my dissertation/research area. I have read statistics that claim new graduate nurses who experience a hostile, non-supportive workplace leave nursing within their first 5 years and do not return. Horizontal violence has become more prevalent, and resolutions must be found. High stress/workload, feelings of lack of support from staff and superiors, and fears for personal safety in the workplace contribute to job dissatisfaction and burnout.

This book is an excellent resource for the management portion of nursing education, organizational efforts to address toxic workplaces, and individuals who are trying to understand the current environment and/or contribute to more positive ones. I believe we can use it to help stop unhealthy patterns and shape workplaces where nurses nurture their young.

Thank you, Beth, for writing such an important work.

Wanda Christie, MNSc, RN, OCN
Assistant Professor of Nursing
Arkansas Tech University
Russellville, AR

Acknowledgments

Anonymous nurses who shared their stories

The stories in *Confident Voices* are based on first-person accounts from nurses who responded to my invitation to talk about their experiences. I have changed identifying information. A huge thank you to all the nurses who shared their experiences with me. They offer powerful learning opportunities that many of us can relate to.

Nurse Book Reviewers

The following nurses reviewed a working draft of this book and offered valuable feedback. I am sincerely grateful for the input from each of these colleagues and know that this book is more a compelling and useful resource because of it. Please note that the reviewers on this list are not necessarily endorsing opinions in this book. It has been a privilege to communicate with each and every one of these colleagues.

Meredith J. Addison, RN, MSN, CEN
Practicing Nurse
Hillsdale, IN

Kathy Black, RN
Clinical Leader
Cardiothoracic/Vascular Surgery
Maine Medical Center
Portland, ME

Cindy Brown, RN, BSN, BC
Director of Nursing
The Merrimack Center, JRI
Tewksbury, MA

Wanda Christie, MNSc, RN, OCN
Assistant Professor of Nursing
Arkansas Tech University, Russellville, AR

Joan Cusack-McGuirk, MA, BSN, NEA-BC
VP & CNO St. Luke's Cornwall Hospital
Newburgh/Cornwall, NY

Nancy Dube, RN, BSed, MPH
School Nurse Consultant
Maine Department of Education
Augusta, ME

Jane Dunstan, MEd, RN, CEN
RN III, Emergency Department Nurse
Newcastle, ME

Durinda K. Durr, RN, MS
Vice president/CNO
Rome Memorial Hospital Rome, NY

Jennifer L. Embree, RN, MSN, CCRN, CCNS, CNABC
Clinical Nurse Specialist
Chief Clinical Officer
Dunn Memorial Hospital
Bedford, IN
Adjunct Faculty, Indiana University School of Nursing, Indianapolis, IN

June Fabre, RN, MBA
Author, *Smart Nursing: Nurse Retention & Patient Safety Improvement Strategies*, 2009, Second Edition, Springer Publishing Company

Julie Forbes, RN
Magnet Coordinator
Oswego Hospital, Oswego, NY

Joy Gorzeman, RN, MSN, MBA
Nurse/Healthcare Administrator
San Marcos, CA

Charlotte Guglielmi, RN, BSN, MA, CNOR
Periopertive Nurse Specialist
Beth Israel Deaconess Medical Center
Boston, MA

Anita M. Hakala, MSN, RN, CNE
Nursing Faculty
Central Maine Medical Center College of Nursing
University of Southern Maine College of Nursing and Healthcare
Professionals
Norway, ME

Meg Helgert, RN, BS, FNP
Portland, OR

Susan Henderson, RN, BS, MA
President of ANA-Maine
Associate Professor Department of Nursing
Saint Joseph's College
Standish, ME

Ellen Horton, RN, MSN
Director of Education/Nursing Institutes
Providence Little Company of Mary Medical Centers-
Torrance/San Pedro, CA

Ellen Interlandi, RN, MHM, NE- BC
Former CNO
Consultant, New Mexico Hospital Association
Board member of the NM Organization of Nurse Executives & the NM
Center for Nursing Excellence
Albuquerque, NM

Karen M. Knapp, RN, BSN, CRNFA
OR Supervisor
Muskegon, MI

Lori Krcatovich, BSN, RN, CNOR, CRNFA
Registered Nurse First Assistant
Holland, MI

Rita Lamy, BSN, RN
Foster Care Health Nurse Coordinator
Manchester District Office

Cindy A. Light, MSN, RN, CEN
Assistant Professor
Baker University, SON, Topeka, KS

Major Suellyn M. Masek, RN, MSN, CNOR
US Army Retired

Cathy O'Malley, RN

Sandra Oswald, RN, BSN, Nurse Educator
Frisbie Memorial Hospital
Rochester, NH

Linda Salvini, RNC, BSN
President of Central Region of the Iowa Nurses Association
Staff Nurse, Des Moines, IA

Anne Sands, RN, MS, CPHQ
Compliance & Risk Manager
York Hospital, York, ME

Jane Smalley, RN, MA, CEN
Nurse Manager ED/CCU
St. Gabriel's Hospital
Little Falls, MN

Barbara Sheff, MA, RN, CPH, HNC
Holistic Nurse and Innkeeper
The Candleshop Inn Bed and Breakfast and Holistic Retreat Center
York Beach, ME

David L. Taylor III, RN MSN, CNOR
Consultant, Perioperative Services
US Army Retired

Helen M. Vialpando, RN, BSN
Director of Surgical Services
Physician's Regional Healthcare System-Collier Boulevard
Naples, FL

Susan K. Wagner, RN, BSN

Laura Webb, RN
Surgical Intensive Care Unit
Durham, NC

Joyce M. Young, RN, BSN
Clinical Manager Central Service/Endoscopy
Danville, KY

Gina M. Zilio-Smith, BSN, RN, OCN, CHPN
Senior Staff Nurse
Gosnell Memorial Hospice House
Scarborough, ME

Contributing authors

Thanks to the many wise leaders I have quoted throughout Confident Voices and to the special contributions by Joan Cusack-McGuirk, Judy Ringer and Wanda Christie.

Special people in my life

For me, the creative processes of writing this book and developing my own confident voice are intricately woven together. I appreciate all of my friends and family who have been so supportive of my work. In addition to my parents and brothers, I am profoundly grateful for the impact that the following people have had on this book and my life.

Curran B. Russell

Pamela Henry

Cheryl Greenfield

Bonnie Kerrick

In addition, I want to thank Diane Brandon, Marilyn Carter, Meg Helgert, Jorinda Margolis, and Nancy Schmid, whose insights, encouragement and friendship have provided wonderful support.

Finally, I am eternally grateful for the input from my publishing team, Jeffrey Elwood, Bonnie Kerrick, and Joanne Muckenhoupt. Each of these professionals has made exceptional contributions to the quality of this publication.

Index

V

W

Y

Z

About the Author and Editor

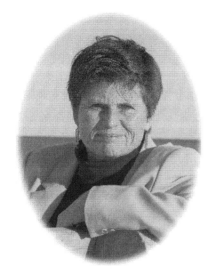

Beth Boynton, RN, MS is a nurse consultant specializing in communication and conflict. She offers a variety of workshops, publishes the free bimonthly eNewsletter: *Confident Voices for Nurses: The Resource for Creating Positive Workplaces*, and numerous articles. She had developed the "Conflict Coach" podcast series for nurse leaders and is a featured columnist for *ANA-Maine Journal*. bbbboynton@earthlink.net.

Bonnie Kerrick, RN, BSN is a former pediatric and community health nurse now practicing as a writer/editor specializing in healthcare and education. Her work includes editing for *Confident Voices for Nurses* eNewsletter and the New York State Museum Magazine, *Legacy*. She is also a grant writer for Strawbery Banke Museum in Portsmouth, NH, and lives in Cape Neddick, Maine, with her husband, Craig. bdk123@maine.rr.com.

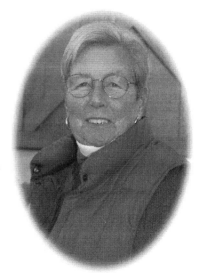

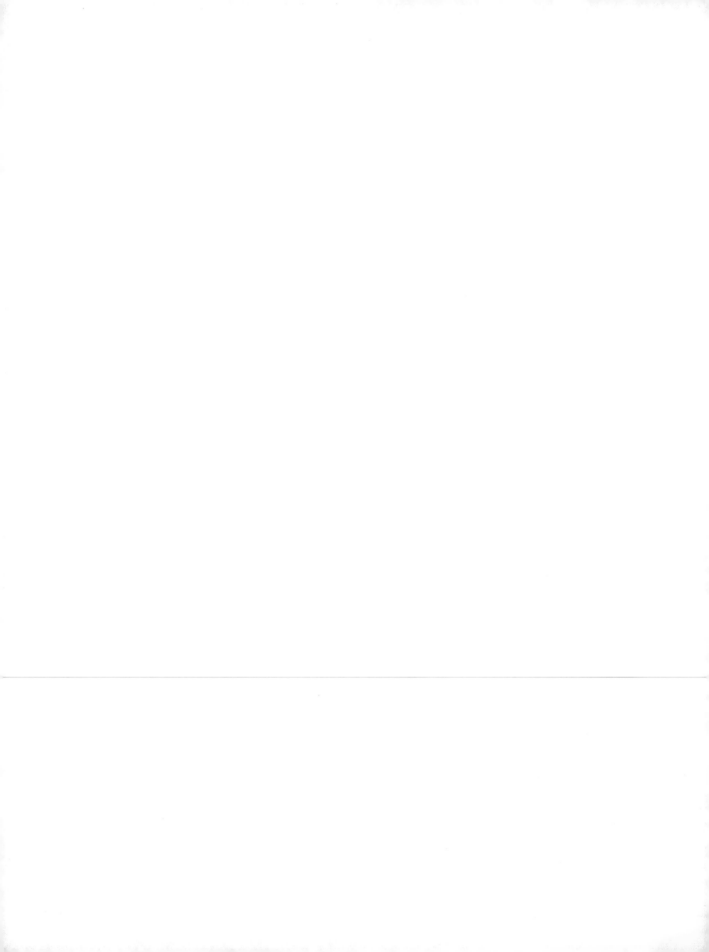

- Notes -

- Notes -

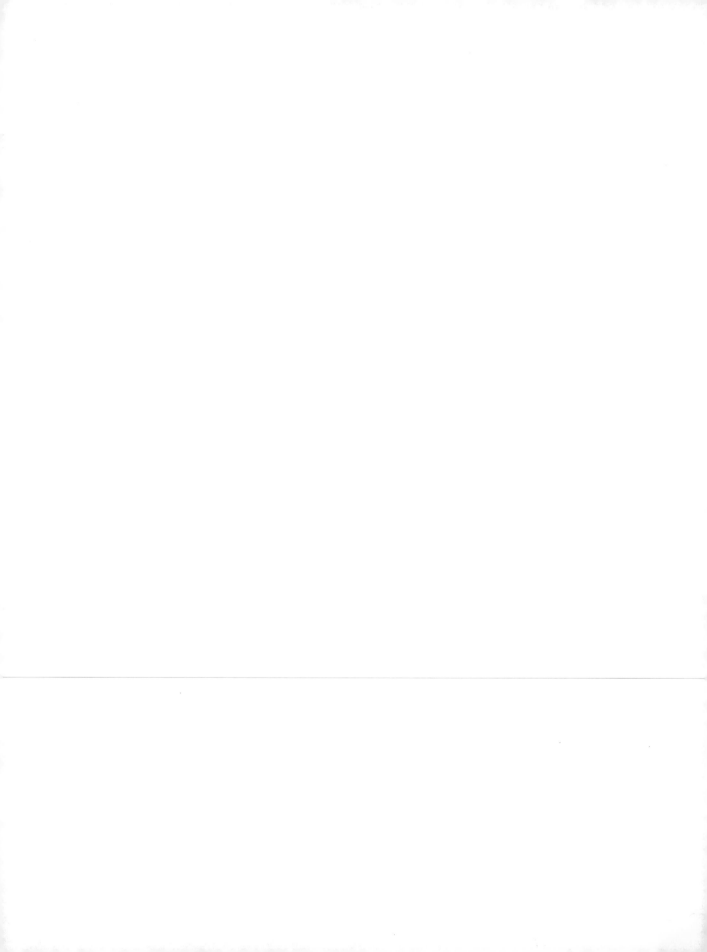

Made in the USA
Lexington, KY
16 November 2013